Current Concepts in Breast Pathology

Guest Editor

LAURA C. COLLINS, MD

SURGICAL PATHOLOGY CLINICS

surgpath.theclinics.com

Consulting Editor
JOHN R. GOLDBLUM, MD

June 2009 • Volume 2 • Number 2

Cover image courtesy of Edi Brogi, MD, PhD and Melissa Murray, DO

SAUNDERS an imprint of ELSEVIER, Inc.

W.B. SAUNDERS COMPANY
A Division of Elsevier Inc.

1600 John F. Kennedy Boulevard • Suite 1800 • Philadelphia, Pennsylvania 19103-2899

http://www.theclinics.com

SURGICAL PATHOLOGY CLINICS Volume 2, Number 2
June 2009 ISSN 1875-9181, ISBN-13: 978-1-4377-0549-2, ISBN-10: 1-4377-0549-9

Editor: Joanne Husovski

Surgical Pathology Clinics (ISSN 1875-9181) is published quarterly by Elsevier Inc., 360 Park Avenue South, New York, NY 10010-1710. Months of issue are March, June, September, and December. Business and Editorial Offices: 1600 John F. Kennedy Blvd., Suite 1800, Philadelphia, PA 19103-2899. Periodicals postage paid at New York, NY and additional mailing offices. Subscription prices are $159.00 per year (US individuals), $199.00 per year (US institutions), $80.00 per year (US students/residents), $199.00 per year (Canadian individuals), $225.00 per year (Canadian Institutions), $199.00 per year (foreign individuals), $225.00 per year (foreign institutions), and $99.00 per year (international & Canadian students/residents). Foreign air speed delivery is included in all *Clinics'* subscription prices. All prices are subject to change without notice. **POSTMASTER:** Send address changes to *Surgical Pathology Clinics*, Elsevier Periodicals Customer Service, 11830 Westline Industrial Drive, St. Louis, MO 63146. Customer Service: 1-800-654-2452 (US). From outside the United States, call 1-314-453-7041. Fax: 1-314-453-5170. E-mail: JournalsCustomerServiceusa@elsevier.com (for print support) and JournalsOnlineSupport-usa@elsevier.com (for online support).

Reprints. For copies of 100 or more, of articles in this publication, please contact the Commercial Reprints Department, Elsevier Inc., 360 Park Avenue South, New York, NY 10010-1710. Tel. (212) 633-3812; Fax: (212) 462-1935; email: reprints@elsevier.com.

Printed in the United States of America.

Contributors

CONSULTING EDITOR

JOHN R. GOLDBLUM, MD
Chairman, Department of Anatomic Pathology,
Cleveland Clinic; and Professor of Pathology,
Cleveland Clinic Lerner College of Medicine,
Cleveland, Ohio

GUEST EDITOR

LAURA C. COLLINS, MD
Associate Director, Division of Anatomic
Pathology, Department of Pathology, Beth
Israel Deaconess Medical Center; and
Assistant Professor of Pathology, Harvard
Medical School, Boston, Massachusetts

AUTHORS

FOUAD I. BOULOS, MD
Department of Pathology, American University,
Beirut, Lebanon

EDI BROGI, MD, PhD
Associate Attending Pathologist, Department
of Pathology, Memorial Sloan-Kettering
Cancer Center, Weill Cornell Medical College,
New York, New York

LAURA C. COLLINS, MD
Associate Director, Division of Anatomic
Pathology, Department of Pathology, Beth
Israel Deaconess Medical Center; and
Assistant Professor of Pathology, Harvard
Medical School, Boston, Massachusetts

ADRIANA D. CORBEN, MD
Clinical Fellow in Pathology, James Homer
Wright Pathology Laboratories of the
Massachusetts General Hospital; and
Department of Pathology, Harvard Medical
School, Boston, Massachusetts

DEBORAH A. DILLON, MD
Assistant Professor, Harvard Medical School;
and Associate Pathologist, Department of
Pathology, Brigham and Women's Hospital,
Boston, Massachusetts

TIMOTHY W. JACOBS, MD
Department of Pathology, Virginia Mason
Medical Center, Seattle, Washington

MELINDA F. LERWILL, MD
Assistant Professor of Pathology, James
Homer Wright Pathology Laboratories of the
Massachusetts General Hospital; and
Department of Pathology, Harvard Medical
School, Boston, Massachusetts

SUSAN C. LESTER, MD, PhD
Assistant Professor, Harvard Medical School;
and Associate Pathologist, Department of
Pathology; and Chief, Breast Pathology
Services, Brigham and Women's Hospital,
Boston, Massachusetts

CHAD A. LIVASY, MD
Associate Professor, Department of Pathology
and Lab Medicine, University of North Carolina,
Chapel Hill, North Carolina

**ANNA MARIE MULLIGAN, MB, MSc,
FRCPath**
Assistant Professor, Anatomic Pathologist,
Department of Laboratory Medicine, St.
Michael's Hospital and University of Toronto,
Toronto, Ontario, Canada

MELISSA MURRAY, DO
Assistant Attending Pathologist, Department
of Pathology, Memorial Sloan-Kettering
Cancer Center, Weill Cornell Medical College,
New York, New York

AYSEGUL A. SAHIN, MD
Department of Pathology, The University
of Texas M. D. Anderson Cancer Center,
Houston, Texas

STUART J. SCHNITT, MD
Director, Division of Anatomic Pathology,
Department of Pathology, Beth Israel
Deaconess Medical Center; and Professor
of Pathology, Harvard Medical School, Boston,
Massachusetts

JEONG YUN SHIM, MD
Department of Pathology, The University
of Texas M. D. Anderson Cancer Center,
Houston, Texas

JEAN F. SIMPSON, MD
Department of Pathology, Vanderbilt University
Medical Center, Nashville, Tennessee

Contents

The correct diagnosis of proliferations within the mammary terminal duct-lobular unit has paramount prognostic and therapeutic implications. Occasionally, the differential diagnosis of compact florid hyperplasia, atypical ductal hyperplasia, and low-grade ductal carcinoma in situ can be quite challenging, with seeming morphologic overlap. This article presents a conceptual and practical understanding of these processes and their impact on subsequent cancer risk, with the intention of assisting the practicing pathologist in rendering accurate and clinically relevant diagnoses for this frequently encountered set of mammary epithelial lesions.

The histopathology, carcinogenesis, clinical behavior, and therapy of triple-negative carcinomas are covered in detail with emphasis on the heterogeneity of this group of tumors. Gene expression profile and immunohistochemical studies of these tumors are discussed including definitions used to define tumors as basal-like. Diagnostic pitfalls are reviewed including immunohistochemical studies valuable in excluding mimics.

Lesions of the breast characterized by enlarged terminal duct lobular units lined by columnar epithelial cells are being increasingly encountered in breast biopsy specimens. Some of these lesions feature cuboidal to columnar epithelial cells in which the lining cells exhibit cytologic atypia. The role of these lesions (recently designated "flat epithelial atypia" [FEA]) in breast tumor progression is still emerging. FEA commonly coexists with well-developed examples of atypical ductal hyperplasia, low-grade ductal carcinoma in situ, lobular neoplasia, and tubular carcinoma. These findings and those of recent genetic studies suggest that FEA is a neoplastic lesion that may represent a precursor to or the earliest morphologic manifestation of ductal carcinoma in situ. Additional studies are needed to better understand the biologic nature and clinical significance of these lesions.

Lobular carcinoma in situ (LCIS) is a heterogeneous disease clinically and morphologically. For many years, LCIS has been regarded as a marker lesion of increased risk for invasive carcinoma. Recent evidence, however, suggests that LCIS represents a nonobligate precursor to invasive carcinoma. The progression of LCIS to invasion appears to be less frequent and slower than for ductal carcinoma in situ

(DCIS). With the application of E-cadherin, pathologists have learned to recognize unusual variants of LCIS that were previously categorized as ductal carcinoma. The appropriate treatment of these special types of LCIS is currently debated as information on the clinical outcome remains very limited at present.

This article focuses on current issues relating to fibroepithelial lesions, predominantly those with cellular stroma, and covers key pathologic features, differential diagnosis, and pitfalls. Phyllodes tumors are emphasized, including the histologic categorization and prognostic features of these lesions. The management of fibroepithelial lesions on needle core biopsy is reviewed.

Papillary lesions of the breast include a broad spectrum of entities, many of which can be diagnostically challenging for the pathologist. This article focuses on encapsulated papillary carcinoma, a recently proposed term used to describe papillary carcinoma occurring within a cystically dilated duct. Previously considered a variant of papillary ductal carcinoma in situ, the finding that these lesions typically lack myoepithelial cells at their periphery has raised questions about their true nature. This article presents a practical approach to the diagnosis of encapsulated papillary carcinoma with a review of its histologic mimics and clinical significance.

Immunohistochemical markers for myoepithelial cells are commonly used to distinguish invasive from noninvasive lesions in the breast. The approach takes advantage of the fact that conventional invasive carcinomas lack surrounding myoepithelial cells, whereas nearly all benign lesions and in situ carcinomas retain their myoepithelial cell layer. Although conceptually straightforward, the interpretation of myoepithelial cell markers can be complicated by misleading patterns of reactivity (such as stromal or tumor cell staining) or lack of reactivity (due to reduced numbers of myoepithelial cells or variable antigenicity). In this article, we discuss the advantages and disadvantages of commonly used myoepithelial cell markers, their general utility in distinguishing invasive from noninvasive processes, and pitfalls in their interpretation. We also examine whether the detection of myoepithelial cells is helpful in the evaluation of papillary lesions, another common application. Myoepithelial cell markers can be diagnostically useful in the distinction of many benign, in situ, and invasive lesions, but they must be interpreted in conjunction with careful morphologic analysis.

Spindle cell lesions of the breast represent a heterogeneous group of reactive and neoplastic disorders that commonly present diagnostic challenges. Arguably, the most important of these lesions to recognize is spindle cell carcinoma, a type of metaplastic carcinoma. This review focuses on those spindle cell lesions of the breast that are most likely to be encountered in clinical practice or that produce particular diagnostic difficulties.

Because of the singular anatomic structure of the nipple, some breast lesions only occur at this site. This article reviews the diagnostic process for such lesions, including squamous metaplasia of lactiferous ducts, duct ectasia, nipple adenoma, large duct papilloma, syringomatous adenoma, Toker cells, and Paget disease of the nipple. Biopsy specimens from these lesions may be small, superficial, or fragmented because of concern about maintaining the cosmetic appearance of the nipple and areola. Knowledge of the location of the biopsy, and the clinical presentation, is often essential in making the correct diagnosis.

Breast lesions associated with extracellular mucin production are uncommon and constitute a wide spectrum of lesions ranging from benign cyst to mucinous carcinoma. Intracytoplasmic mucin can be seen rarely in benign metaplasias but is a common finding in invasive and in situ carcinomas. In this article, we discuss the differential diagnosis of breast lesions associated with mucin production and other entities that show histologic changes that mimic mucin production.

Surgical Pathology Clinics

FORTHCOMING ISSUES

Current Concepts in Gastrointestinal Pathology
John Hart, MD and Amy Noffsinger, MD,
Guest Editors

Current Concepts in Gynecologic Pathology
Esther Oliva, MD, *Guest Editor*

Current Concepts in Dermatopathology
Steven Billings, MD, *Guest Editor*

RECENT ISSUES

Current Concepts in Genitourinary Pathology: Kidney and Testes
Anil V. Parwani, MD, PhD, *Guest Editor*

Current Concepts in Genitourinary Pathology: Prostate and Bladder
Anil V. Parwani, MD, PhD, *Guest Editor*

THE CLINICS ARE NOW AVAILABLE ONLINE!

Access your subscription at:
www.theclinics.com

Preface

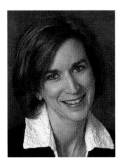

Laura C. Collins, MD
Guest Editor

Breast pathology can be challenging for all of us involved in diagnostic surgical pathology. Several areas of breast pathology are particularly difficult or problematic. Breast pathology is the focus of this issue of the *Surgical Pathology Clinics* series, and experts in the field have provided comprehensive reviews of commonly encountered problematic lesions in breast pathology, including proliferative epithelial lesions, fibroepithelial lesions, mucinous lesions, and spindle cell lesions. Additionally, this issue includes a state-of-the-art review of the use of myoepithelial markers in the differential diagnosis of benign, in situ, and invasive lesions, a differential diagnostic situation that many of us encounter daily. Finally, there is an article covering the topic of triple-negative breast cancers, a subtype of breast cancer that has garnered much interest in recent years because of the overlap with the recently described molecular subtype of basal-like breast cancers.

In each article, high-quality photomicrographs complement the text where appropriate to further illustrate the relevant points. In addition, each article reviews the key features and differential diagnostic considerations of the lesions being discussed and highlights potential pitfalls to avoid.

It is hoped that the reviews presented in this issue of the *Surgical Pathology Clinics* will be a useful resource to all pathologists involved in diagnostic breast pathology.

Laura C. Collins, MD
Associate Director
Division of Anatomic Pathology
Beth Israel Deaconess Medical Center
Assistant Professor of Pathology
Harvard Medical School
330 Brookline Avenue
Boston, MA 02215, USA

E-mail address:
lcollins@bidmc.harvard.edu

doi:10.1016/j.path.2009.02.007
1875-9181/09/$ – see front matter

DIFFERENTIAL DIAGNOSIS OF PROLIFERATIVE BREAST LESIONS

Jean F. Simpson, MD[a],*, Fouad I. Boulos, MD[b]

KEYWORDS

• Epithelial proliferative disease • Ductal carcinoma in situ

ABSTRACT

The correct diagnosis of proliferations within the mammary terminal duct-lobular unit has paramount prognostic and therapeutic implications. Occasionally, the differential diagnosis of compact florid hyperplasia, atypical ductal hyperplasia, and low-grade ductal carcinoma in situ can be quite challenging, with seeming morphologic overlap. This article presents s conceptual and practical understanding of these processes and their impact on subsequent cancer risk, with the intention of assisting the practicing pathologist render accurate and clinically relevant diagnoses for this frequently encountered set of mammary epithelial lesions.

PROLIFERATIVE BREAST LESIONS

OVERVIEW

Epithelial proliferations within the terminal duct-lobular unit (TDLU), including usual patterns of hyperplasia and atypical ductal hyperplasia (ADH), are commonly encountered breast lesions. The correct classification of these proliferations carries significant implications for the subsequent risk of developing invasive cancer. Most examples of usual or ordinary patterns of hyperplasia, ADH, and ductal carcinoma in-situ (DCIS) pose little diagnostic challenge for practicing pathologists. For cases that seem to be borderline, careful application of diagnostic criteria allows assignment into the appropriate category. In general, the authors' approach for borderline cases is to favor the lesser diagnosis.

A general understanding of the formative elements of proliferative lesions is necessary for proper classification. These fundamental principles include location, pattern and extent of spread, and cellular morphology. Immunohistochemical studies have little application in this differential diagnosis. This article focuses on the diagnostic criteria for usual patterns of hyperplasia, ADH, and low-grade DCIS, with practical guidelines for diagnosing borderline lesions encountered either on core biopsy or in excision specimens.

GROSS FEATURES

In general, the proliferative breast lesions described in this article do not present grossly detectable alterations. Exuberant examples of ordinary hyperplasia as well as some examples of low-grade DCIS may, rarely, form a mass when the specimen is examined grossly. Far more information is gained by a careful review of the specimen imaging studies, with attention to correlating tissue sectioning with imaging findings. The regular absence of noticeable gross changes supports complete submission of the tissue when practical. For specimens too large for complete submission, an ex vivo radiograph of tissue slices can guide sampling.

[a] Department of Pathology, Vanderbilt University Medical Center, C-3318 Medical Center North, Nashville, TN 37232, USA
[b] Department of Pathology, American University, Beirut, Lebanon
* Corresponding author.
E-mail address: jean.simpson@vanderbilt.edu (J.F. Simpson).

Surgical Pathology 2 (2009) 235–246
doi:10.1016/j.path.2009.02.002
1875-9181/09/$ – see front matter

surgpath.theclinics.com

Key Features
PROLIFERATIVE BREAST LESIONS

Usual hyperplasia without atypia

1. Cellular features: variability, nuclear overlap, uneven cell placement, indistinct cell borders

2. Architecture: peripheral secondary spaces, cellular swirling patterns, thin tapering cellular bars

3. Extent: usually involves a single TDLU but may be more extensive

Atypical ductal hyperplasia

1. Cellular features: cellular monotony and uniformity; even placement of small cells

2. Architecture: rigid secondary spaces, crisp cribriform spaces, and rigid arching bars

3. Extent: incomplete involvement of spaces, residual normal polarized epithelium

DCIS (low grade)

1. Cellular features: cellular monotony and uniformity, even placement of small cells

2. Architecture: rigid secondary spaces, crisp cribriform spaces, and rigid arching bars

3. Extent: complete involvement of two adjacent spaces, often involves true duct, usually larger than 3 mm

Pitfalls
PITFALLS IN THE DIAGNOSIS OF PROLIFERATIVE BREAST LESIONS

! Thick histologic sections create the appearance of cellular monotony.

! Gynecomastoid pattern of usual hyperplasia mimics micropapillary ADH or DCIS.

! Papillary apocrine change may mimic micropapillary ADH or DCIS.

! ADH involving enlarged lobular units may suggest DCIS because of its size.

! In collagenous spherules the crisp spaces mimic ADH.

! Solid pattern of ADH may mimic lobular neoplasia.

! The fragmented nature of core biopsy precludes assessment of the extent of disease.

MICROSCOPIC FEATURES

Usual patterns of hyperplasia as well as ADH and low-grade DCIS are located within the TDLU. Usual hyperplasia is often termed "ordinary" to underscore that this pattern is the one found most frequently in benign breast biopsies. Usual hyperplasia is characterized by a proliferation of bland, variably sized cells in a streaming, swirling, or jumbled arrangement with nuclear overlap. The cells lack distinct cell borders. The nuclei usually are oval or carrot-shaped instead of round, may contain grooves and "helioid" inclusions, but lack conspicuous nucleoli (**Fig. 1**). As the cells proliferate, the residual lumen of the involved space becomes peripheral and compressed (**Fig. 2**). The proliferating cells form irregular bridges, and tethered tufts are often present. The degree of involvement does not change the

assignment of this pattern of proliferation to the usual or ordinary category. The architecture of the proliferation within the involved space is a result of the relationship that the proliferating cells have with one another. The overlapping cells of usual-pattern hyperplasia result in thin, irregularly tapered tufts and bridges (**Figs. 3–5**). Frequently, cellular bars seem to consist of strands of anuclear cytoplasm. One pattern of ordinary hyperplasia resembles that of gynecomastia, with mounds of pyknotic cells heaped on underlying luminal epithelium (**Fig. 6**).

ADH is defined in terms of its resemblance to low-grade DCIS, but a critical distinction is the extent of involvement. ADH is characterized by a proliferation of monomorphic cells that are evenly spaced. This even placement results in secondary spaces that appear "rigid" or static, rather than the "fluid" streaming and swirling of usual-pattern hyperplasia. ADH is composed of a uniform population of bland cells with round nuclei and distinct cell borders. Architecturally, ADH can be solid, cribriform, micropapillary, or a combination thereof. The cribriform spaces are crisply round and regular, and the cellular bridges are rigid (**Fig. 7**). The cells of micropapillary ADH form bulbous projections composed of the same monomorphic cells that partially line the involved space; the micropapillae have narrow stalks that interdigitate with the luminal cells.

The distinction between ADH and low-grade DCIS depends on the extent of involvement within

Fig. 1. Usual hyperplasia without atypia. Note the cellular variability, uneven cell placement, and irregular secondary spaces. Several "helioid" inclusions are present.

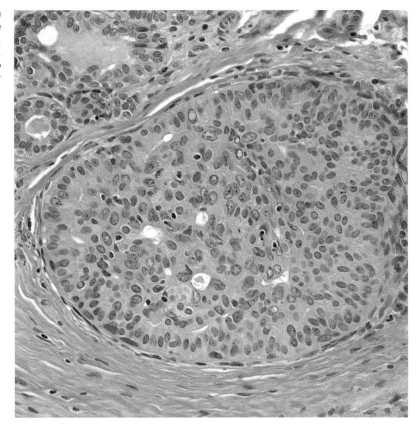

Fig. 2. Usual hyperplasia without atypia. This terminal ductal lobular unit contains usual-pattern hyperplasia. As the cells proliferate, the resulting secondary spaces are peripheral and slitlike. Note the swirling arrangement of the proliferating cells and their indistinct cell borders.

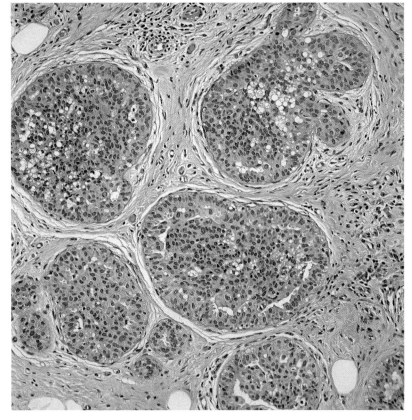

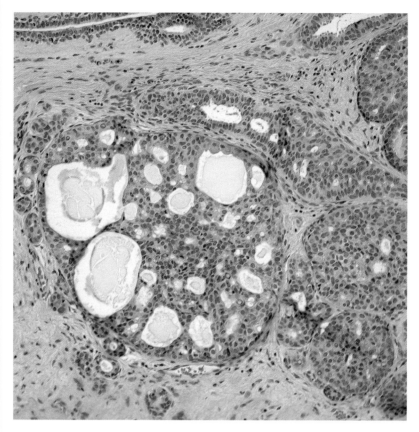

Fig. 3. Usual hyperplasia without atypia. At first glance, the secondary spaces appear regular, but close examination shows cellular bars composed of cells that are not uniform in appearance or in placement. Note the thin, tapering strand of cytoplasm that separates the two larger secondary spaces at left.

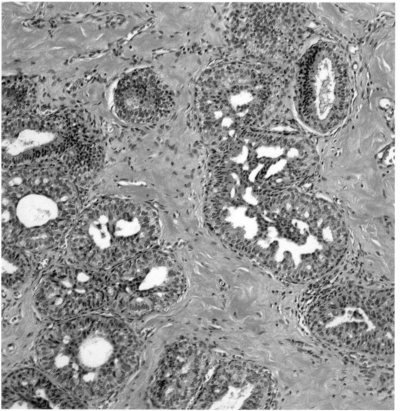

Fig. 4. Irregular cellular bars identify this example as usual hyperplasia without atypia.

Fig. 5. The cellular bars that define secondary spaces are thin, delicate, and tapering, all features of usual hyperplasia; some are composed of wisps of anuclear cytoplasm.

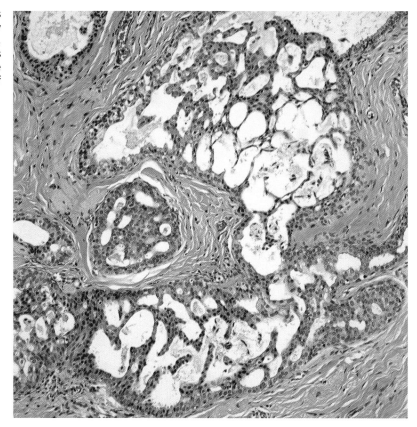

Fig. 6. This partially involved space contains tapering projections of proliferating cells that appear "stuck" on the underlying luminal epithelium. This pattern is seen in gynecomastia and in the female breast is part of usual hyperplasia without atypia.

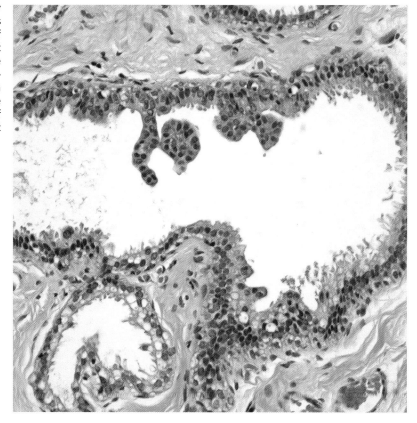

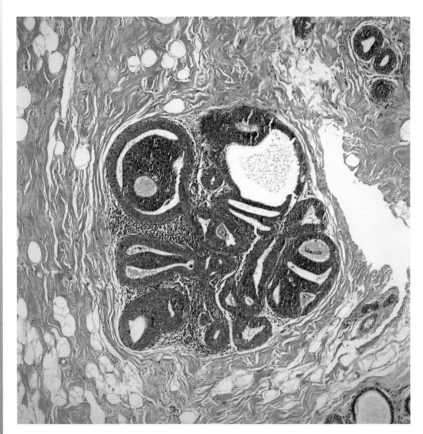

Fig. 7. Atypical ductal hyperplasia. This TDLU contains a population of uniform, evenly spaced cells that are arranged in rigid cellular bars. None of the spaces is replaced completely by the neoplastic cells, thus negating a diagnosis of DCIS.

the TDLU. DCIS is diagnosed when the characteristic uniform population of cells completely fills two adjacent spaces; any lesser involvement is, by definition, ADH (**Fig. 8**). As a matter of practicality, DCIS is usually at least 3 mm in extent; smaller lesions are better categorized as ADH. That statement, however, does not mean that any monomorphic proliferation larger than 3 mm is DCIS; partial involvement of unfolded, enlarged lobular units qualifies as ADH (**Fig. 9**). Another helpful feature is that DCIS usually involves true ducts (**Fig. 10**). Usually DCIS completely involves multiple spaces, namely expanded and unfolded lobular units and intervening ducts.

The diagnostic principles relating to low-grade lesions cease to apply when the neoplastic cell population shows advanced cytologic atypia. In the presence of advanced cytologic atypia (often in the presence of necrosis), a diagnosis of DCIS can be made on a single partially involved space, with the certainty that more extensive disease will be present in additional sections or in the excision specimen that follows the diagnostic biopsy. The salient diagnostic features of proliferative breast lesions are summarized in the key Features Box.

DIFFERENTIAL DIAGNOSIS

In general terms, the differential diagnosis for ordinary hyperplasia is ADH, which in turn must be distinguished from low-grade DCIS. The differential diagnosis for DCIS includes unusual patterns of invasive carcinoma known as "invasive cribriform carcinoma."

Usual patterns of hyperplasia, when presenting a solid growth pattern, can be confused with ADH or low-grade DCIS (see **Fig. 3**). Making the correct diagnosis is facilitated by thin microscopic sections. Thick sections give the illusion of cellular monotony. Attention to cellular variability and overlap will assure the correct diagnosis. When usual hyperplasia resembles the pattern present in gynecomastia, it can mimic micropapillary ADH or even DCIS. This pattern is characterized by mounds of cells with pyknotic nuclei that seem to be "stuck" on luminal cells (see **Fig. 6**).

Fig. 8. Low-grade DCIS, cribriform type. The changes are sufficient to diagnose DCIS because two adjacent spaces are completely populated by the neoplastic cell population. In this example, a smaller space at bottom is involved also. The overall size of this area is 3 mm.

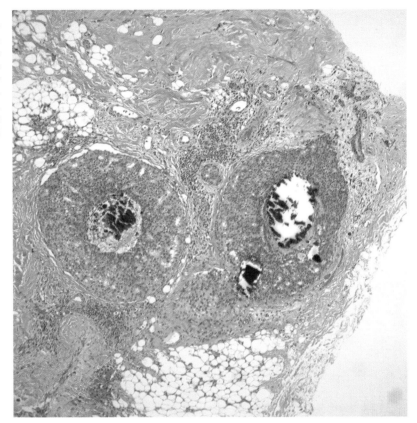

Fig. 9. Several spaces within this unfolded and enlarged lobular unit are partially involved by a uniform population of cells with rigid architecture. Although the overall size of this area is 5 mm, ADH is diagnosed because of partial involvement.

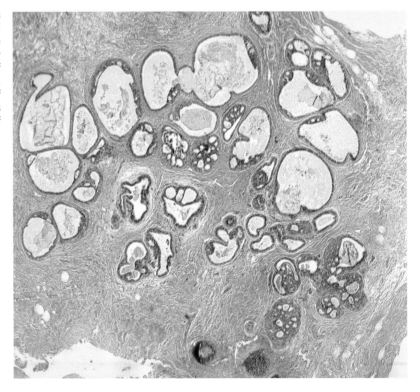

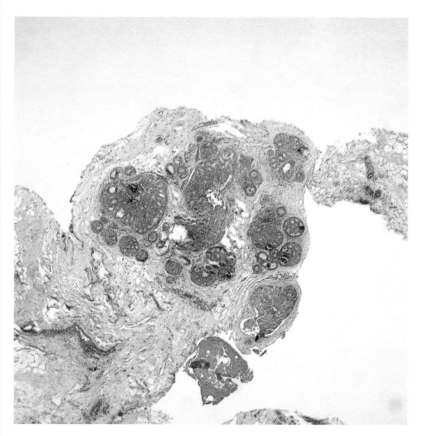

Cellular uniformity and crisp, regular secondary spaces are the diagnostic clues to ADH. ADH is a spatially limited, predominantly lobulocentric, low-grade and low-volume atypical proliferation that does not have the ability to involve and unfold a TDLU completely or to spread to other TDLUs across duct systems. When these features are completely present in two adjacent basement membrane–bound spaces, DCIS is diagnosed. DCIS usually involves true ducts and extends over an area of 3 to 4 mm (**Fig. 11**). It is important to remember that the differential diagnostic alternative for ADH is low-grade DCIS; intermediate- or high-grade DCIS is diagnosed even when present in lesser extent.

Some have advocated the use of immunohistochemical studies to distinguish ordinary patterns of hyperplasia from ADH. In an effort to improve diagnostic agreement in proliferative breast lesions, MacGrogan and colleagues[1] used immunohistochemical analysis for CK5/6 and E-cadherin in a series of 105 cases. Generally speaking the diagnostic agreement based on morphologic grounds was moderate and was not improved

significantly using these immunohistochemical markers.

Collagenous spherulosis is an uncommon finding within the breast, and its clinical significance is not known. The presence of true lumens and "pseudolumens" that contain basement membrane material occasionally can be confused with the crisp, rigid secondary spaces of ADH or DCIS (**Fig. 12**). Recognizing the two different types of spaces may be aided by the use of a periodic acid-Schiff alcian blue stain.

Occasionally lobular neoplasia (either atypical lobular hyperplasia or lobular carcinoma in situ) may be confused with TDLU involvement by solid pattern ADH or DCIS. A careful search for distinct cell–cell borders and microrosettes helps the clinician arrive at the proper diagnosis. Immunohistochemical expression of E-cadherin may be helpful in this distinction, with the realization that there may be aberrant expression.[2]

Invasive cribriform carcinoma is an uncommon form of breast carcinoma that occasionally can be confused with cribriform-type DCIS (**Fig. 13**). Careful attention to the lack of a lobulocentric

Fig. 11. Higher magnification of Fig. 10, showing involvement of a true duct at the bottom.

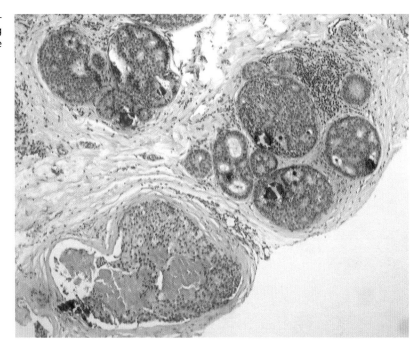

Fig. 12. Collagenous spherulosis mimics ADH with seeming crisp secondary spaces. Closer inspection shows the presence of true lumens and pseudolumens; the latter contain basement membrane material.

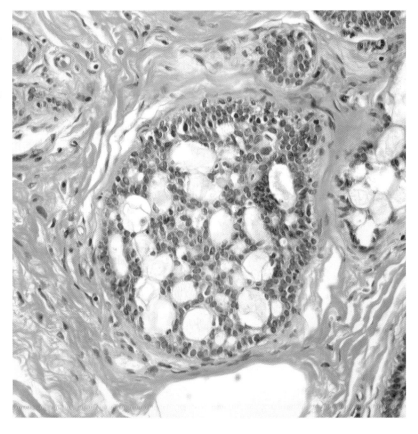

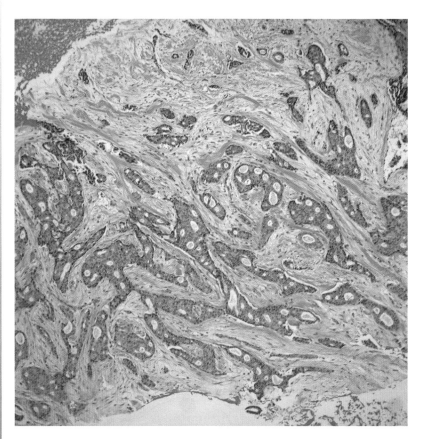

Fig. 13. Invasive cribriform carcinoma. Although the individual islands resemble cribriform DCIS, the infiltrative nature and lack of lobulocentricity characterize this lesion as an invasive carcinoma. Invasive cribriform carcinoma is biologically analogous to tubular carcinoma.

process and the absence of a myoepithelial cell layer helps identify the invasive nature of this form of invasive carcinoma, which has an excellent prognosis.

DIAGNOSIS ON CORE BIOPSY

If ordinary patterns of hyperplasia are diagnosed on core biopsy, and there is concordance with imaging studies, further excision is not necessary.

A number of studies report clinically significant diagnostic upgrades in the excisional biopsy specimen after a diagnosis of ADH on core biopsy, and thus excision is the usual recommendation in this setting. In an extensive review of the literature, the gauge of the biopsy device and the size of the lesion were the statistically significant factors that reduced underestimation at the time of core biopsy.[3] Using an 11-gauge vacuum-assisted device, Sohn and colleagues[4] were able to reduce by half the often-quoted upgrade rate of 36%. Even though needle core biopsies may excise the lesion completely, the nature of the procedure presents a fragmented specimen, precluding an assessment of the extent of

involvement, which is critical in the distinction between ADH and low-grade DCIS. Quantification of ADH within core biopsies has been attempted to predict the presence (or absence) of more advanced disease within the excisional biopsy specimen.[5] Upgrades are more likely if there are more than two foci of ADH, if the lesion is larger than 6 mm, or if the lesion is smaller than 6 mm but is not removed completely.[6] This finding is not surprising, because low-grade DCIS usually is at least 4 mm in extent. It does point out, however, that small, limited disease could be spared formal excision. It is likely that the practice of excising ADH detected on core biopsy will continue, based on the characteristics of the specimen obtained by the majority of needle biopsy devices currently in use. The authors maintain a conservative approach in borderline cases, diagnosing ADH and recommending excision to evaluate the full extent of the lesion. This approach allows the definitive diagnosis to be made on excision, without subjecting the patient to unnecessary additional therapy for a lesion amenable to cure by adequate surgery alone.

If ADH is present within an excisional biopsy specimen, no further surgical intervention is

Table 1
Relative risk associated with proliferative breast disease: Nashville Breast Cohort

Lesion	Increase in Relative Risk	Laterality of Risk
Usual patterns of hyperplasia	1.5–2 times	Bilateral risk
Atypical ductal hyperplasia	4–5 times	Bilateral risk
Low-grade DCIS	9–10 times	Ipsilateral risk

Data from Dupont W, Page D. Risk factors for breast cancer in women with proliferative breast disease. N Engl J Med 1985;312:146–51; and Page DL, Dupont WD, Rogers LW, et al. Continued local recurrence of carcinoma 15–25 years after a diagnosis of low grade ductal carcinoma in situ of the breast treated only by biopsy. Cancer 1995;76:1197–200.

necessary. In general, the finding of ADH at a margin of an excisional biopsy is of no consequence, unless it is at the periphery of an area of DCIS. The decision for re-excision should take the imaging findings into consideration: if no imaged abnormality remains, re-excision may not be necessary.

CLINICAL IMPLICATIONS AND PROGNOSIS

The relative risks associated with various proliferative lesions are shown in **Table 1**. Note that ordinary or usual hyperplasia and ADH are associated with bilateral risk, whereas low-grade DCIS carries a risk of ipsilateral breast cancer. A number of large epidemiologic studies[7–9] have confirmed the original work of Dupont and Page[10] (**Table 2**).

From a practical point of view, the risk associated with ordinary-pattern hyperplasia is insufficient (1.5 times increased risk) to affect patient management. The diagnosis of ADH is associated with an increased relative risk of subsequent breast cancer development 4 to 5 times that in age-matched controls.[10] Although ADH is a well-established risk indicator, the implications for an individual patient are less certain. Some women receive screening mammograms more frequently, but this approach is not proven or universally accepted.

The subsequent bilateral risk associated with ADH is significantly different from the risk associated with low-grade DCIS and is evidence that ADH is not an obligate precursor for in situ or invasive carcinoma. Thus, the diagnostic distinction of ADH from low-grade DCIS has important therapeutic implications. There is some molecular evidence indicating that ADH shares genetic alterations with more advanced lesions,[11] but long-term follow-up studies characterizing ADH at the molecular level in the absence of more advanced lesions are not available.

The natural history of low-grade non-comedo DCIS is one of progression to invasive cancer over a period that may extend over many years.[12] From the Nashville Breast Cohort, Page and colleagues[12] retrospectively identified 28 cases of low-grade DCIS initially diagnosed as benign. In long-term follow-up, nine women developed invasive carcinoma, all in the breast in which the original DCIS was found (and in same site, when documented). It is important to remember that these DCIS lesions were detected in the era before mammography and were present in specimens removed for some non-DCIS palpable abnormality. Furthermore, no attempt at clear margins was undertaken. It therefore is sound to consider DCIS a nonobligate precursor that has a significant likelihood of progression if not excised completely. The Nurses' Health Study has provided additional support for the understanding of the natural history

Table 2
Confirmatory studies of proliferative breast disease: increase in relative risk

Pathologic Finding	Nashville Breast Cohort (1985)[10]	Nurses' Health Study (1992)[7]	Breast Cancer Detection Demonstration Project (1993)[8]	Mayo Clinic (2005)[9]
Usual hyperplasia without atypia	1.5–2 times	1.6 times	1.3 times	1.9 times
Atypical ductal hyperplasia	4–5 times	3.7 times	4.3 times	4.2 times

of DCIS as a precursor to invasive carcinoma. In a review of 1877 cases, 13 cases originally diagnosed as benign were reclassified as DCIS.[13] Six women developed invasive carcinoma, all in the ipsilateral breast. Similar to the findings of Page and colleagues,[12] some of the cancers developed many (up to 18) years after the initial biopsy that, in retrospect, contained DCIS; this development was especially the case for low-grade DCIS.[13]

The objective of current therapeutic strategies is to curtail this natural evolution without sacrificing the whole breast. More recent studies have shown that the three most important determinants of recurrence/progression are the histologic characteristics of the DCIS, its size, and its margin status.[14] These three elements have been used to create the Van Nuys Prognostic Index (VNPI) that predicts the likelihood of disease recurrence. A recent review of 215 patients who underwent breast conservation surgery for DICS (without additional radiotherapy or hormonal therapy) showed that the presence of comedo necrosis and the VNPI were the only significant factors in predicting disease recurrence.[15]

In summary, specific histologic criteria for proliferative lesions of the breast have been linked to outcome through large epidemiologic studies. Careful application of these criteria will continue to identify women who are at an increased risk for later development of cancer and those whose risk is no greater than that in age-matched controls.

REFERENCES

1. MacGrogan G, Arnould L, de Mascarel I, et al. Impact of immunohistochemical markers, CK5/6 and E-cadherin on diagnostic agreement in non-invasive proliferative breast lesions. Histopathology 2008;52:689–97.

2. DaSilva L, Parry S, Reid L, et al. Aberrant expression of E-cadherin in lobular carcinomas of the breast. Am J Surg Pathol 2008;32:773–83.

3. Houssami N, Ciatto S, Ellis I, et al. Underestimation of malignancy of breast core-needle biopsy. Cancer 2007;109:487–95.

4. Sohn V, Arthurs Z, Herbert G, et al. Atypical ductal hyperplasia: improved accuracy with the 11-gauge vacuum-assisted versus the 14-gauge core biopsy needle. Ann Surg Oncol 2007;14(9):2497–501.

5. Ely K, Carter BA, Jensen RA, et al. Core biopsy of the breast with atypical ductal hyperplasia: a probabilistic approach to reporting. Am J Surg Pathol 2001;25:1017–21.

6. Forgeard C, Benchaib M, Guerin N, et al. Is surgical biopsy mandatory in case of atypical ductal hyperplasia on 11-gauge core needle biopsy? A retrospective study of 300 patients. Am J Surg 2008; 196:339–45.

7. London S, Connolly JL, Schnitt SJ, et al. A prospective study of benign breast disease and the risk of breast cancer. JAMA 1992;267:941–4.

8. Dupont W, Parl FF, Hartmann WH, et al. Breast cancer risk associated with proliferative breast disease and atypical hyperplasia. Cancer 1993;71: 1258–65.

9. Hartmann L, Sellers TA, Frost MH, et al. Benign breast disease and the risk of breast cancer. N Engl J Med 2005;353:229–37.

10. Dupont W, Page D. Risk factors for breast cancer in women with proliferative breast disease. N Engl J Med 1985;312:146–51.

11. Lakhani S, Collins N, Stratton MR, et al. Atypical ductal hyperplasia of the breast: clonal proliferation with loss of heterozygosity on chromosomes 16q and 17p. J Clin Pathol 1995;48:611–5.

12. Page D, Dupont WD, Rogers LW, et al. Continued local recurrence of carcinoma 15–25 years after a diagnosis of low grade ductal carcinoma in situ of the breast treated only by biopsy. Cancer 1995; 76:1197–200.

13. Collins LC, Tamimi RM, Baer HJ, et al. Outcome of patients with ductal carcinoma in situ untreated after diagnostic biopsy: results from the nurses' health study. Cancer 2005;103(9):1778–84.

14. Guerra LE, Smith RM, Kaminski A, et al. Invasive local recurrence increased after radiation therapy for ductal carcinoma in situ. Am J Surg 2008; 196(4):552–5.

15. Gilleard O, Goodman A, Cooper M, et al. The significance of the Van Nuys Prognostic Index in the management of ductal carcinoma in situ. World J Surg Oncol 2008;6:61.

TRIPLE-NEGATIVE BREAST CARCINOMA

Chad A. Livasy, MD

KEYWORDS

- Breast cancer • Triple-negative breast cancer • Basal-like • Estrogen receptor • BRCA1

ABSTRACT

Triple-negative breast carcinomas (TNBCs) comprise approximately 15% to 20% of breast cancers. Accurate assessment of tumor estrogen receptor, progesterone receptor, and human epidermal growth factor receptor 2 (HER2) status is an essential part of classifying tumors into this group. As a group, these tumors are associated with poor clinical outcomes and have been shown to exhibit an increased propensity for hematogenous metastasis to the brain and lungs. Many TNBCs, particularly ductal, not otherwise specified (NOS), and metaplastic carcinomas, show an overlapping characteristic gene expression pattern when evaluated by cDNA microarrays. This group has been termed basal-like because of the similarity with normal breast basal/myoepithelial cells including basal cytokeratin expression and lack of hormone receptor and HER2 expression. The array data have been used to develop multiple immunohistochemical surrogates to identify basal-like tumors in formalin-fixed, paraffin-embedded tissues, most employing basal cytokeratins and epidermal growth factor receptor. Currently, there is no international consensus on biomarkers used to identify tumors as basal-like, and the routine use of the term basal-like in surgical pathology reports is premature. Tumor morphologic features associated with triple-negative status include Nottingham grade 3 with high mitotic rate, pushing border of invasion, geographic tumor necrosis, solid/sheet-like growth pattern, lymphocytic infiltrate, and large central acellular zone. Most breast cancers arising in patients who have a germ-line BRCA1 mutation show similar histologic features and a triple-negative phenotype. Not all TNBCs are associated with an unfavorable prognosis, drawing attention to the heterogeneity of this tumor group and the continued need to link tumor morphology and grade with triple-negative status. This article focuses on histopathology, molecular characterization, carcinogenesis, clinical behavior, and treatment of these tumors.

Interest in estrogen receptor-negative, progesterone receptor-negative, HER2-negative, "triple-negative" invasive breast cancers has increased because of multiple factors, including a better understanding of the diversity of breast cancer. Over the past 10 years. there has been increasing recognition that breast cancer is a heterogeneous disease, diverse in natural history and responsive to treatments. This understanding has been facilitated by the evolution of gene expression profiling of tumors and the development of a molecular classification of breast cancers. It is known that variations in tumor gene expression account for much of the biologic diversity observed in breast cancer. Molecular studies of breast tumors have identified multiple intrinsic subtypes of breast cancer, each showing a characteristic gene expression pattern.[1–3] These groupings include both hormone receptor-positive subtypes called luminal (A or B), and at least two hormone receptor-negative subtypes designated basal-like and HER2. The basal-like and HER2 subtypes are associated with poor clinical outcomes. The triple-negative breast carcinomas (TNBCs) show significant overlap with the basal-like cancers, but these terms are not synonymous. The term triple-negative is based on immunohistochemical or in situ assays for estrogen receptor (ER), progesterone receptor (PR), and HER2, while the term basal-like is based on the cDNA microarray gene expression pattern.

The success of HER2-targeted therapy observed in several clinical trials for HER2-positive tumors has spurred further interest in TNBCs in an attempt to find effective targeted therapy for these tumors.

Department of Pathology and Lab Medicine, University of North Carolina, CB# 7525 Brinkhous-Bullitt Building, Chapel Hill, NC 27599-7525, USA
E-mail address: cal@med.unc.edu

Surgical Pathology 2 (2009) 247–261
doi:10.1016/j.path.2009.02.005
1875-9181/09/$ – see front matter

From the oncologist's perspective, there are three general groups of breast cancer: hormone receptor-positive tumors where endocrine therapy plays a major role in treatment, HER2-positive tumors where HER2-targeted therapy plays a major role in therapy, and triple-negative tumors where chemotherapy is the mainstay of treatment. Unlike other tumor subtypes, effective targeted therapy agents do not exist for TNBCs. The main utility in grouping the TNBCs together, particularly ductal, NOS and metaplastic carcinomas, is to focus research on identifying the mechanisms of carcinogenesis for these tumors and to develop effective novel therapies through clinical trials.

GROSS FEATURES

TNBCs show a range of variation in their gross appearance. These tumors have an increased propensity to show a more circumscribed gross appearance when compared with hormone receptor-positive tumors (**Fig. 1**). When these well circumscribed spherical tumors present in young women, they can be confused with fibroadenoma on physical examination and mammographic studies. Due in large part to the high proliferative rate of most of these tumors, the average presenting tumor size for triple-negative tumors is larger than that observed for hormone receptor-positive tumors. Triple-negative tumors are more likely to present as interval tumors compared with hormone receptor-positive tumors. The cut surface of these tumors ranges from tan to gray/white and may

Key Features
HISTOLOGIC FINDINGS ASSOCIATED WITH TRIPLE-NEGATIVE PHENOTYPE

Grade 3 histology with high mitotic rate

Pushing margin of invasion

Focal geographic tumor necrosis

Lymphocytic stromal response

Medullary features

Solid/sheet-like growth pattern

Ribbon-like growth pattern

Large central zone of fibrosis/necrosis

Metaplastic features

Myoepithelial differentiation

Salivary gland differentiation

Apocrine differentiation

Secretory differentiation

show varying degrees of necrosis. The necrotic foci often appear yellow or red/brown when associated with hemorrhage. Some variants show extensive central necrosis or a large central fibrotic zone.

MICROSCOPIC FEATURES

TNBCs show tremendous diversity in their histopathologic appearance. The most common

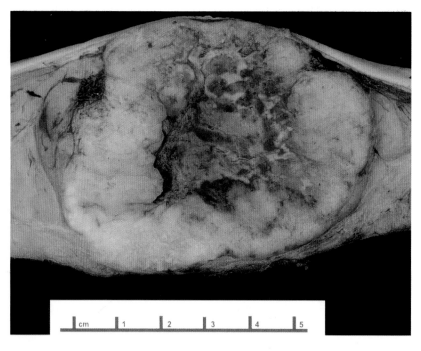

Fig. 1. Macroscopic example of a large triple-negative breast carcinoma with pushing margins and central zone of hemorrhagic necrosis. Multiple smaller punctate foci of yellow necrosis are seen in the more peripheral aspects of the tumor.

TNBCs are ductal, NOS carcinomas, and many of these tumors show some overlapping histopathologic features. Microscopic features most frequently observed in ductal NOS carcinomas with a triple-negative phenotype include grade 3 histology, pushing margin, lymphoid stroma, comedo necrosis, and central fibrosis/necrosis (**Fig. 2**).[4] Not surprisingly, many of these histopathologic features overlap with those described as associated with invasive basal-like breast cancers. Histologic features associated with basal-like breast cancers identified by gene microarray analysis include markedly elevated mitotic rate ($P<0.0001$), geographic tumor necrosis ($P<0.0001$), pushing margin of invasion ($P=0.0001$), and lymphocytic response ($P=0.01$).[5] Many

Fig. 2. Histologic features of ductal, NOS carcinomas with triple-negative phenotype include pushing margin of invasion (*A*), lymphoplasmacytic inflammatory response at the margin of the tumor (*B*).

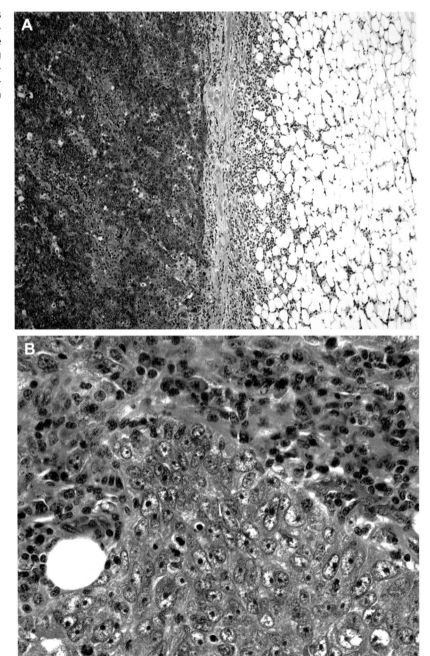

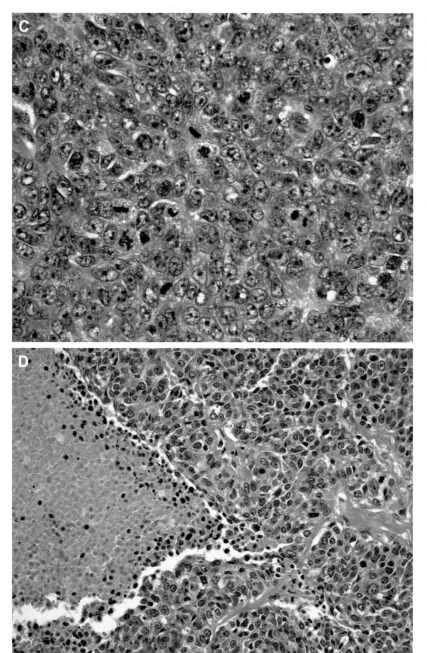

Fig. 2. Grade 3 histology including solid/sheet-like architecture and markedly elevated mitotic index (*C*), foci of geographic necrosis (*D*).

triple-negative ductal NOS carcinomas also show tumor cells with high nuclear/cytoplasmic ratios, solid/sheet-like architecture pattern, and a syncytial arrangement of tumor cells. The constellation of findings in several of these tumors is similar to those previously used to describe atypical medullary carcinomas, a term that has fallen out of favor because of the lack of favorable prognosis associated with these tumors.[6] Other less common architectural patterns associated with triple-negative status include large, central fibrotic acellular zone and ribbon-like architecture associated with central necrosis (see **Fig. 2**). Tsuda and colleagues[7,8] have described a series of

Fig. 2. Large central acellular fibrotic zone (*E*), and ribbon-like architecture associated with large zone of central comedo necrosis (*F*).

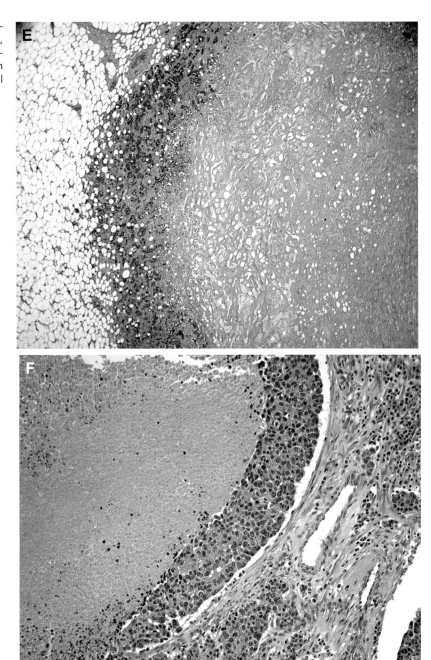

high-grade invasive ductal carcinomas with large, central acellular zones showing aggressive clinical behavior and myoepithelial differentiation. In the author's experience, tumors with this morphology frequently show a triple-negative phenotype.

Metaplastic carcinomas show marked diversity in their histopathologic features and are almost exclusively triple-negative. These unusual tumors comprise approximately 1% of all breast cancers.

Most of these tumors show an admixture of high-grade adenocarcinoma and dominant areas of spindled/sarcomatoid, squamous, matrix-producing, chondroid, or osteoid differentiation (**Fig. 3**). Rare low-grade variants of metaplastic carcinoma exist, including low-grade adenosquamous carcinoma and low-grade spindle cell carcinoma, both often exhibiting a triple negative phenotype.

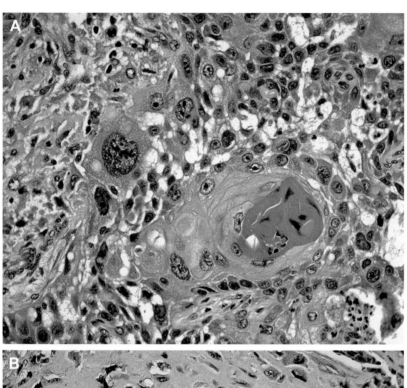

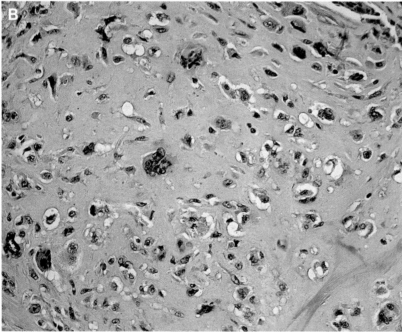

Fig. 3. High-grade metaplastic carcinomas show diverse histopathology including squamous differentiation, occasionally with squamous pearl formation (*A*), chondroid differentiation (*B*).

✱ Other rare histologic variants of invasive breast carcinoma associated with triple-negative phenotype include adenoid cystic carcinoma, apocrine carcinoma, myoepithelial carcinoma, and secretory carcinoma (**Fig. 4**). Tumors showing apocrine differentiation in greater than 90% of the tumor, including eosinophilic granular cytoplasm with large nuclei, vesicular chromatin, and prominent nucleoli are almost always hormone receptor-negative, but not necessarily triple-negative. A significant subset of these tumors, approximately 50%, will show HER2 overexpression, with the

Fig. 3. Osteoid differentiation (*C*), and spindled/sarcomatoid differentiation (*D*). The quantity of admixed adenocarcinoma with these tumors is highly variable.

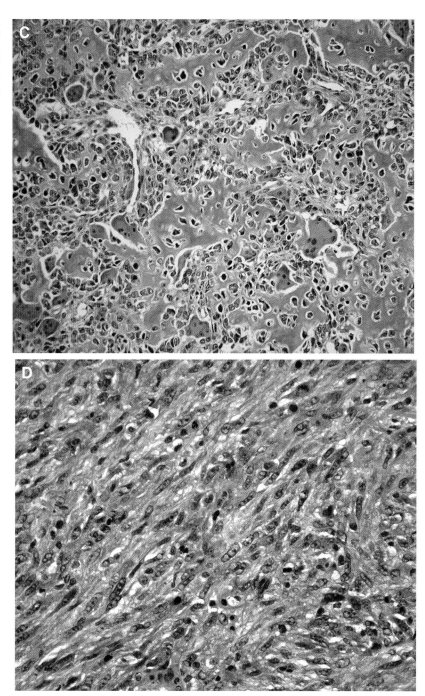

remainder being triple-negative. Myoepithelial carcinomas and adenoid cystic carcinomas are essentially always triple-negative, indicative of their non-luminal cell of origin. Myoepithelial carcinomas (malignant myoepithelioma) typically are characterized by a proliferation of infiltrating spindle cells with minimal-to-mild nuclear atypia, low-grade mitotic activity (less than 3 to 4 mf/10 hpf), and immunoreactivity for smooth muscle actin, calponin, and S100. Primary breast adenoid cystic carcinomas show histology very similar to those seen in the salivary gland, including a biphasic proliferation of epithelial cells with predominance of basaloid cells arranged in cribriform and tubular formations. A few of these tumors show increased solid architecture and

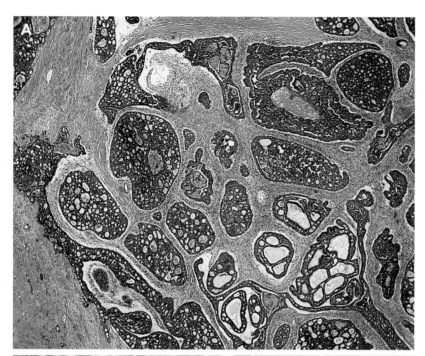

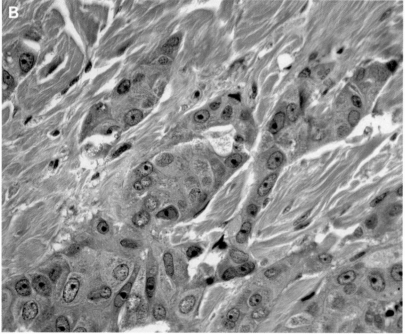

Fig. 4. Rare histologic subtypes of breast cancer associated with triple-negative phenotype include adenoid cystic carcinoma (*A*), apocrine carcinoma (*B*).

necrosis, which some have reported to be associated with more aggressive clinical behavior. Secretory carcinomas are characterized by marked secretory changes including eosinophilic vacuolated cytoplasm and prominent intra- and extra-cellular eosinophilic secretions, usually located within the lumen of tubules. Secretory carcinomas show variable receptor findings, but most of these tumors demonstrate a triple-negative phenotype.

Fig. 4. Myoepithelial carcinoma (*C*), and secretory carcinoma (*D*).

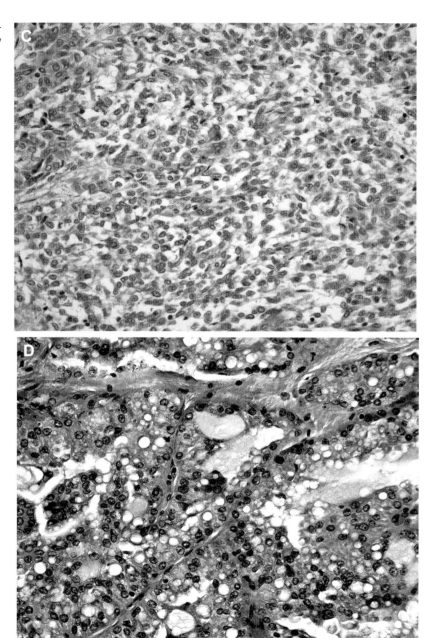

Most BRCA1-associated invasive breast cancers show a triple-negative phenotype by immunohistochemistry and a basal-like subtype by gene expression profiling.[3,9–12] BRCA1-associated breast cancers frequently show a common constellation of histopathologic features including tumor circumscription, sheet-like growth pattern, lymphoid infiltrate, high mitotic rate, prominent nucleoli, and necrosis.[13] These observations indicate that the morphology and receptor status of a breast cancer can assist in the triaging of patients for BRCA1 genetic testing. Attention to the histologic features of a patient's breast cancer can improve selection criteria for genetic testing, thus improving sensitivity to detect BRCA1 mutations. Farshid and colleagues[13] demonstrated that morphology could predict the likelihood of association with a BRCA1 mutation in a series of breast cancers with a sensitivity of 92%, specificity of 86%, positive predictive value of 61%, and negative predictive value of 98%. Documentation of high-risk morphologic features in pathology reports of young women who have breast cancer could be particularly useful in triaging patients who have small families or limited family history knowledge.

DIFFERENTIAL DIAGNOSIS

The diagnosis of most TNBCs is typically straightforward. Because of the lack of differentiation in some of these tumors, including complete absence of tubule formation, the differential diagnosis in some cases includes diffuse large B-cell lymphoma, metastatic poorly differentiated carcinoma, malignant melanoma, and sarcoma. Difficulty in excluding these other neoplasms on morphology alone is exaggerated on core biopsies with limited sampling of the tumor. The diffuse solid growth pattern of large cell lymphoma may resemble some of the poorly differentiated TNBCs, but the neoplastic lymphocytes typically show less striking nuclear atypia with small-to-absent nucleoli and increased cellular discohesion compared with carcinomas. Immunohistochemical stains for pan-cytokeratin, CD20, and CD3 easily distinguish these entities.

Metastatic carcinoma should be considered in patients who have a history of carcinoma elsewhere, multiple nonpalpable breast lesions on mammography, and absence of in situ carcinoma component in biopsy specimens. Lung non-small cell carcinomas, including those with neuroendocrine differentiation, are the most common tumors to metastasize to the breast and may show histologic features similar to poorly differentiated ductal or metaplastic carcinomas. Immunohistochemical studies may be of limited utility, as poorly differentiated lung non-small cell carcinomas and TNBCs are often negative for TTF1 and GCDFP-15, respectively. Interpretation of the histopathologic findings in the clinical and radiographic context is essential in excluding metastasis. Another problematic scenario is when a poorly differentiated triple-negative carcinoma presents in an axillary lymph node, and the corresponding breast mammographic studies are negative. The differential diagnosis in these cases involves occult breast, lung, head and neck, and occasionally gynecologic primaries. Identification of the primary site may not be possible in all cases. The presence of papillary architecture and psammoma bodies raises suspicion of a serous adenocarcinoma of gynecologic primary.

Spindle-cell metaplastic carcinomas, depending on nuclear grade, may show similar histopathologic features to sarcoma (high nuclear grade) or fibromatosis (low nuclear grade). The most likely diagnosis for every sarcomatous-appearing lesion in the breast is metaplastic carcinoma. Focal epithelioid features are present in most high-grade sarcomatoid metaplastic carcinomas. A panel of high and low molecular weight cytokeratins is recommended in these lesions to evaluate for epithelial differentiation. Primary breast sarcomas that may mimic certain TNBCs include epithelioid angiosarcoma and undifferentiated postradiation sarcoma. Distinction of low-grade metaplastic spindle cell carcinoma from fibromatosis is more problematic. This distinction is often not possible on a core biopsy specimen. An immunohistochemical panel of broad-spectrum cytokeratins and p63 is recommended for these cases. Low-grade spindle cell carcinomas may show only focal weak immunoreactivity for these markers.

DIAGNOSIS

GENE EXPRESSION PROFILING STUDIES

Results of gene expression profiling studies of 42 breast cancers published by Perou and colleagues[1] in 2000 identified a subtype of breast cancer termed basal-like because of its similarity to the expression pattern observed in normal breast basal/myoepithelial cells. The other breast cancer subtypes identified in the original publication include luminal, normal breast-like, and HER2. The basal-like carcinomas showed expression of basal cytokeratins 5 and 17, epidermal growth factor receptor (EGFR), c-KIT, and proliferation genes (including Ki-67 and PCNA) and down-regulation of ER, PR, and HER2 expression. Knowledge of the gene expression profile of these tumors, including decreased ER/PR/HER2 expression, has been used to devise immunohistochemical surrogate assays to identify basal-like cancers in archived formalin-fixed, paraffin-embedded tissues. The details of these assays are discussed in the following section. Although most TNBCs cluster with the basal-like subtype,

---

▲▲ Differential Diagnosis

Large cell lymphoma

Granulocytic sarcoma

Metastatic carcinoma

Metastatic melanoma

Epithelioid angiosarcoma

Undifferentiated sarcoma

Malignant phyllodes tumor

Fibromatosis

there is up to 30% discordance between immunohistochemical- and microarray-defined subtypes.[14–17] Gene microarray analysis remains the current gold standard for determining breast cancer subtype, including those classified as basal-like. It is important to remember that the molecular subtypes identified to date are based primarily on ductal, NOS carcinomas. Expression profiling results on rare triple-negative tumors including adenoid cystic carcinoma and low-grade metaplastic carcinomas have not been reported. Other molecular subtypes are likely to be identified in the future as more breast cancers undergo gene expression profiling.

IMMUNOHISTOCHEMISTRY

A tremendous number of studies have addressed the immunohistochemical profile of triple-negative and basal-like breast cancers. The definitions and nomenclature used in these studies are inconsistent and have led to confusion about classification of both triple-negative and basal-like breast cancers. The author has identified tumors showing a lack of HER2 overexpression or amplification with ER and PR Allred scores of 0 or 2 as triple-negative. Rare tumors are difficult to classify showing weak ER and PR expression (1% to 5% nuclear positivity) or borderline HER2 amplification (HER2:CEP17 1.8-2.2). Accurate assessment of tumor ER, PR, and HER2 status is essential in correctly classifying tumors into the triple-negative group. Attention to preanalytic factors (details of fixation time and fixative), method of antigen retrieval, and antibody clone used is needed to ensure accurate results.

Surrogate immunohistochemical studies to define tumors as basal-like have used different criteria to define a tumor as basal-like. These studies have demonstrated significant immunophenotypic heterogeneity among these tumors. Suffice it to say that there is no internationally accepted standard on biomarkers used to identify a tumor as basal-like, and the routine use of the term basal-like in pathology reports is premature. The identification of basal cytokeratin expression in triple-negative tumors is confirmatory of a basal-like subtype, but not all basal-like carcinomas demonstrate positivity for basal cytokeratins by immunohistochemistry.[1–3,5,17–19] The most widely used immunohistochemical surrogate to define a tumor as basal-like is that proposed by Nielsen and colleagues,[17] where basal-like carcinomas were defined as those lacking ER and HER2 expression and expressing cytokeratin 5/6 and/or EGFR. This four-biomarker panel demonstrated a sensitivity of 76% and a specificity of 100%. Many other biomarkers are reported to be associated with basal-like carcinoma and are listed in **Box 1**.[20–31] Because of the scarcity of fresh tumor for gene expression profiling, interest in surrogate immunohistochemical panels to define tumor subtype will persist for the near future. Quantitative RT-PCR based assays someday may play a role in determining tumor subtypes, as these assays are becoming more standard on formalin-fixed, paraffin-embedded tissues.

CARCINOGENESIS AND EPIDEMIOLOGY

Little is known about the carcinogenesis of TNBCs. TNBCs are a diverse group of tumors with multiple mechanisms of carcinogenesis. A subset of these tumors arising in carriers of germ-line BRCA1 mutations shows consistent morphologic features and basal-like subtype indicating a link between the mechanism of carcinogenesis and tumor phenotype. Given that several sporadic breast cancers show a similar phenotype and subtype by gene expression profiling, BRCA1 dysfunction also may play a role in the pathogenesis of sporadic basal-like breast cancers. Studies have shown lower BRCA1 mRNA expression in

---

Box 1
Biomarkers with reported increased expression in basal-like carcinomas

Basal cytokeratins (cytokeratins 5, 14 and 17)

Epidermal growth factor receptor (EGFR)

Vimentin

Smooth muscle proteins (smooth muscle actin, calponin)

p63

Laminin

Maspin

Nestin

Fascin

P-cadherin

Cyclin E

Nerve growth factor receptor (NGFR)

c-KIT

Vascular endothelial growth factor (VEGF)

Caveolin-1

αβ-crystallin

β4 integrin

Proliferation-associated proteins (Ki-67 and PCNA)

basal-like breast cancers compared with matched controls.[32] Knowledge of the mechanism of carcinogenesis for TNBCs, such as defective DNA repair mechanisms, someday may play a role in the selection of therapeutic agents.

Epidemiologic studies shave shown increased prevalence of triple-negative and basal-like breast cancers among premenopausal African American women.[33–35] Risk factors reported to be associated with basal-like tumors include parity combined with lack of breast feeding, early-onset menarche, younger age at first full-term pregnancy, elevated waist-hip ratio, and gain in adiposity since childhood.[33] Women with multiple live births who did not breast feed and women who used medication to suppress lactation were at increased risk for basal-like breast cancer. Some of the associations, including increased risk for parity and younger age at first full-term pregnancy, were opposite those observed for the luminal (hormone receptor-positive) tumors. Longer duration breast feeding, increasing number of children breast fed, and increasing number of months breast feeding per child were each associated with reduced risk of basal-like breast cancer.

PROGNOSIS

Several studies have shown inferior prognosis associated with triple-negative and basal-like breast cancers, particularly when compared with hormone receptor-positive tumors.[2,3,33,36,37] TNBCs have been shown to have an increased likelihood of distant recurrence and death within 5 years of diagnosis. Dent and colleagues[36] studied 1601 patients who had breast cancer and found that the risk of distant recurrence in TNBCs peaked around 3 years and declined rapidly thereafter. In contrast, hormone receptor-positive tumors showed a recurrence risk that seemed to be constant over the period of follow-up. Other observations from their study of triple-negative tumors include a weak relationship between tumor size and node status, distant recurrence rarely preceded by local recurrence, local recurrence not predictive of distant recurrence, and rapid progression from distant recurrence to death.

Other studies have shown uniqueness to the patterns of metastasis and relapse for TNBCs.[37,38] Triple-negative tumors consistently show more aggressive visceral disease (eg, lung) and soft tissue disease, and less common bone relapse, when compared with hormone receptor-positive tumors. Triple-negative tumors also have been shown to be over-represented in patients who have brain metastasis. In one study of over 3000 patients, triple-negative status was the greatest risk factor for the developing cerebral metastasis.[39]

TNBCs are a heterogeneous group of tumors, and they include rare histologic subtypes showing a more favorable prognosis. Oncologists may be unaware of the relatively more favorable prognosis associated with adenoid cystic carcinoma, low-grade spindle cell carcinoma, low-grade adenosquamous carcinoma, and secretory carcinoma. It is important to clarify the prognostic significance of these histologic subtypes in the pathology report, emphasizing the continued need to interpret triple-negative status in the context of tumor grade and histology.

Although triple-negative phenotype generally is associated with poor clinical outcomes, these tumors show sensitivity to chemotherapy. Chemotherapy has been the mainstay of treatment for these tumors, as effective targeted therapies are currently unavailable. Both adjuvant and neoadjuvant studies have shown higher sensitivity of

Pitfalls

! The solid sheet-like growth pattern of some large cell lymphomas and granulocytic sarcoma may mimic a poorly differentiated TNBC, particularly when tumor sampling is scant in a core biopsy. Immunohistochemistry using pan-cytokeratin, CD20, CD3, and CD45 typically resolves this differential diagnosis easily.

! Metastatic carcinomas involving the breast, particularly of lung, thymic, head and neck, or gynecologic primary, may mimic TNBC. Clinical history of prior malignancy, multiple (often nonpalpable) breast masses, absence of an in situ component, and atypical histology should raise suspicion of metastasis.

! High-grade sarcomas including epithelioid angiosarcoma and undifferentiated sarcoma may mimic high-grade metaplastic breast carcinoma. Most metaplastic carcinomas have focal epithelioid features, and the epithelial differentiation can be confirmed with pan-cytokeratin cocktail immunostain.

! Fibromatosis shows significant histologic overlap with low-grade spindle cell breast carcinoma. Excision of the entire mass often is required along with battery of immunostains for high and low molecular weight cytokeratins and p63. Immunoreactivity for these antibodies may be only focal and weak in low-grade spindle cell carcinoma.

TNBCs to anthracycline and anthracycline/taxane-based regimens compared with hormone receptor-positive tumors.[40,41] TNBCs show a significantly higher rate of pathologic complete response to neoadjuvant chemotherapy as compared with hormone receptor-positive tumors. Although TNBCs appear to be more sensitive to neoadjuvant chemotherapy than ER-positive tumors, higher relapse rates are observed among tumors not completely eradicated by chemotherapy.[41,42] Disease-free survival and overall survival remain lowest among the triple-negative and ER-/PR-/HER2+ breast cancers. These findings highlight the need for novel therapies for TNBCs.

Studies have shown that tumors with BRCA1 dysfunction are sensitive to agents that cause DNA damage, such as cisplatin and carboplatin. Knowledge of the association between BRCA1 dysfunction and triple-negative phenotype has led to several studies demonstrating activity of platinum-based regimens for treating TNBCs.[43,44] Clinical trials are underway evaluating several targeted therapies for TNBCs, including poly (ADP-ribose) polymerase (PARP) inhibitors, EGFR-targeted agents, and antiangiogenic agents.[45–52] Hopefully continued focus on this group of tumors in clinical trials will lead to effective targeted therapies with minimal adverse effects, such as those that have been developed for HER2-positive tumors.

REFERENCES

1. Perou CM, Sorlie T, Eisen MB, et al. Molecular portraits of human breast tumours. Nature 2000; 406:747–52.

2. Sorlie T, Perou C, Tibshirani R, et al. Gene expression patterns of breast carcinomas distinguish tumor subclasses with clinical implications. Proc Natl Acad Sci U S A 2001;98:10869–74.

3. Sorlie T, Tibshirani R, Parker J, et al. Repeated observation of breast tumor subtypes in independent gene expression data sets. Proc Natl Acad Sci U S A 2003;100:8418–23.

4. Putti TC, Abd El-Rahim DM, Rakha EA, et al. Estrogen receptor-negative breast carcinomas: a review of morphology and immunophenotypical analysis. Mod Pathol 2005;18:26–35.

5. Livasy CA, Karaca G, Nanda R, et al. Phenotypic evaluation of the basal-like subtype of invasive breast carcinoma. Mod Pathol 2006;19:264–71.

6. Gaffey MJ, Mills SE, Frierson HF, et al. Medullary carcinoma of the breast: interobserver variability in histopathologic diagnosis. Mod Pathol 1995;8:31–8.

7. Tsuda H, Takarabe T, Hasegawa F, et al. Large, central acellular zones indicating myoepithelial tumor differentiation in high-grade invasive ductal

carcinomas as markers of predisposition to lung and brain metastases. Am J Surg Pathol 2000;24: 197–202.

8. Tsuda H, Takaarabe T, Hasegawa T, et al. Myoepithelial differentiation in high-grade ductal carcinomas with large central acellular zones. Hum Pathol 1999;30:1134–9.

9. Foulkes WE, Brunet JS, Stefaansson IM, et al. The prognostic implication of the basal-like (cyclin E high/p27 low/p53+/glomeruloid-microvascular proliferation+) phenotype of BRCA1-related breast cancer. Cancer Res 2004;64:356–62.

10. Vazri SA, Krumroy LM, Elson P, et al. Breast tumor immunophenotype of BRCA1-mutation carriers is influenced by age at diagnosis. Clin Cancer Res 2001;7:1937–45.

11. Foulkes WD, Stefansson IM, Chappuis PO, et al. Germline BRCA1 mutations and a basal epithelial phenotype in breast cancer. J Natl Cancer Inst 2003;95:1482–5.

12. Lakhani M, Loman N, Borg A, et al. Prediction of BRCA1 status in patients with breast cancer using estrogen receptor and basal phenotype. Clin Cancer Res 2005;11:5175–80.

13. Farshid G, Balleine RL, Cumming M, et al. Morphology of breast cancer as a means of triage of patients for BRCA1 genetic testing. Am J Surg Pathol 2006;30:1357–66.

14. Bertucci F, Finetti P, Cervera N, et al. How basal are triple-negative breast cancers? Int J Cancer 2008; 123:236–40.

15. Cleator S, Heller W, Coombes R. Triple-negative breast cancer: therapeutic options. Lancet Oncol 2007;3:235–44.

16. Kreike B, van Kouwenhove M, Horlings H, et al. Gene expression profiling and histopathological characterization of triple-negative/basal-like breast carcinomas. Breast Cancer Res 2007;9:R65.

17. Nielsen T, Hsu F, Jensen K, et al. Immunohistochemical and clinical characterization of the basal-like subtype of invasive breast carcinoma. Clin Cancer Res 2004;10:5367–74.

18. van de Rijn M, Perou CM, Tibshirani R, et al. Expression of cytokeratins 17 and 5 identifies a group of carcinomas associated with poor clinical outcome. Am J Pathol 2002;161:1991–6.

19. Abd El-Rehim DM, Pinder SE, Paish CE, et al. Expression of basal and luminal cytokeratins in human breast carcinoma. J Pathol 2004;203:661–71.

20. Rodriguez-Pinilla SM, Sarrio D, Honrado E, et al. Vimentin and laminin expression is associated with basal-like phenotype in both sporadic and BRCA1-associated breast carcinomas. J Clin Pathol 2007; 60:1017–23.

21. Tsuda H, Morita D, Kimura M, et al. Correlation of KIT and EGFR overexpression with invasive ductal carcinoma of the solid-tubular subtype, nuclear

grade 3, and mesenchymal or myoepithelial differentiation. Cancer Sci 2005;96:48–53.

22. Diaz LK, Cristofanilli M, Zhou X, et al. Beta4 integrin subunit gene expression correlates with tumor size and nuclear grade in early breast cancer. Mod Pathol 2005;18:1165–75.

23. Matos I, Dufloth R, Alvarenga M, et al. p63, cytokeratin 5, and P-cadherin: three molecular markers used to distinguish basal phenotype in breast carcinomas. Virchows Arch 2005;447:688–94.

24. Arnes JB, Brunet JS, Stefansson I, et al. Placental cadherin and the basal epithelial phenotype of BRCA1-related breast cancer. Clin Cancer Res 2005;11:4003–11.

25. Ribeiro-Silva A, Ramalho LN, Garcia SB, et al. p63 correlates with both BRCA1 and cytokeratin 5 in invasive breast carcinomas: further evidence for the pathogenesis of the basal phenotype of breast cancer. Histopathology 2005;47:458–66.

26. Koker MM, Kleer CG. p63 expression in breast cancer: a highly sensitive and specific marker of metaplastic carcinoma. Am J Surg Pathol 2004;28:1506–12.

27. Li H, Cherukuri P, Li N, et al. Nestin is expressed in basal/myoepithelial layer of the mammary gland and is a selective marker of basal epithelial breast tumors. Cancer Res 2007;67:501–10.

28. Reis-Filho JS, Steele D, Palma S, et al. Distribution and significance of nerve growth factor receptor (NGFR/p75NTR) in normal, benign, and malignant breast tissue. Mod Pathol 2006;19:307–19.

29. Reis-Filho JS, Milanezi F, Silva P, et al. Maspin expression in myoepithelial tumors of the breast. Pathol Res Pract 2001;197:817–21.

30. Moyano JV, Evans JR, Chen F, et al. AlphaB-crystallin is a novel oncoprotein that predicts poor clinical outcome in breast cancer. J Clin Invest 2006;116:261–70.

31. Pinilla SM, Honrado E, Hardisson D, et al. Caveolin-1 expression is associated with a basal-like phenotype in sporadic and hereditary breast cancer. Breast Cancer Res Treat 2006;99:85–90.

32. Turner NC, Reis-Filho JS, Russell AM, et al. BRCA1 dysfunction in sporadic basal-like breast cancer. Oncogene 2007;26:2126–32.

33. Carey L, Perou C, Livasy C, et al. Race, breast cancer subtypes, and survival in the Carolina Breast Cancer Study. JAMA 2006;295:2492–502.

34. Bauer K, Brown M, Cress R, et al. Descriptive analysis of estrogen receptor (ER)-negative, progesterone receptor (PR)-negative, and HER2-negative invasive breast cancer, the so-called triple-negative phenotype: a population-based study from the California Cancer Registry. Cancer 2007;109:1721–8.

35. Morris G, Naidu S, Topham A, et al. Differences in breast carcinoma characteristics in newly diagnosed African-American and Caucasian patients: a single-institution compilation compared with the National Cancer Institute's surveillance, epidemiology, and end results database. Cancer 2007;110:876–84.

36. Dent RTM, Pritchard KI, Hanna WM, et al. Triple-negative breast cancer: clinical features and patterns of recurrence. Clin Cancer Res 2007;13:4429–34.

37. Liedtke C, Mazouni C, Hess K, et al. Response to neoadjuvant therapy and long-term survival in patients with triple-negative breast cancer. J Clin Oncol 2008;26:1275–81.

38. Smid M, Wang Y, Zhang Y, et al. Subtypes of breast cancer show preferential site of relapse. Cancer Res 2008;68:3108–14.

39. Heitz F, Harter P, Traut A, et al. Cerebral metastases (CM) in breast cancer (BC) with focus on triple-negative tumors. J Clin Oncol 2008;26 [Abstract 1010].

40. Hayes N, Thor A, Dressler L, et al. HER2 and response to paclitaxel in node-positive breast cancer. N Engl J Med 2007;357:1496–506.

41. Carey L, Dees E, Sawyer L, et al. The triple negative paradox: primary tumor chemosensitivity of breast cancer subtypes. Clin Cancer Res 2007;13:2329–34.

42. Rouzier R, Perou C, Symmans W, et al. Breast cancer molecular subtypes respond differently to preoperative chemotherapy. Clin Cancer Res 2005;11:5678–85.

43. Sirohi B, Arnedos M, Popat S, et al. Platinum-based chemotherapy in triple-negative breast cancer. Ann Oncol 2008;19:1847–52.

44. Yi S, Uhm J, Cho E, et al. Clinical outcomes of metastatic breast cancer patients with triple-negative phenotype who received platinum-containing chemotherapy [abstract]. J Clin Oncol 2008;26.

45. Carey L, Mayer E, Marcom P, et al. TBCRC 001: EGFR inhibition with cetuximab in metastatic triple negative (basal-like) breast cancer [abstract]. Breast Cancer Res Treat 2007;106.

46. Garber J, Richardson A, Harris L, et al. Neo-adjuvant cisplatin (CDDP) in triple-negative breast cancer (BC) [abstract]. Breast Cancer Res Treat 2006;100.

47. O'Shaughnessy J, Weckstein D, Vukelja S, et al. Preliminary results of a randomized phase II study of weekly irinotecan/carboplatin with or without cetuximab in patients with metastatic breast cancer [abstract]. Breast Cancer Res Treat 2007;106.

48. Carey LA, Rugo HS, Marcom PK, et al. TBCRC 001: EGFR inhibition with cetuximab added to carboplatin in metastatic triple-negative (basal-like) breast cancer [abstract]. J Clin Oncol 2008;26.

49. Bryant H, Schultz N, Thomas H, et al. Specific killing of BRCA2-deficient tumours with inhibitors of poly(ADP-ribose) polymerase. Nature 2005;434:913–7.

50. Farmer H, McCabe N, Lord CJ, et al. Targeting the DNA repair defect in BRCA mutant cells as a therapeutic strategy. Nature 2005;434:917–21.

51. Kopetz S, Mita MM, Mok I, et al. First in human phase I study of BSI-201, a small molecule inhibitor of poly ADP-ribose polymerase (PARP) in subjects with advanced solid tumors [abstract]. J Clin Oncol 2008;26.

52. Miller K, Wang M, Gralow J, et al. Paclitaxel plus bevacizumab versus paclitaxel alone for metastatic breast cancer. N Engl J Med 2007;357: 2666–76.

FLAT EPITHELIAL ATYPIA OF THE BREAST

Laura C. Collins, MD

KEYWORDS
- Breast • Columnar cell • Flat epithelial atypia • Low-grade neoplasia

ABSTRACT

L esions of the breast characterized by enlarged terminal duct lobular units lined by columnar epithelial cells are being encountered increasingly in breast biopsy specimens. Some of these lesions feature cuboidal to columnar epithelial cells in which the lining cells exhibit cytologic atypia. The role of these lesions (recently designated "flat epithelial atypia" [FEA]) in breast tumor progression is still emerging. FEA commonly coexists with well-developed examples of atypical ductal hyperplasia, low-grade ductal carcinoma in situ, lobular neoplasia, and tubular carcinoma. These findings and those of recent genetic studies suggest that FEA is a neoplastic lesion that may represent a precursor to or the earliest morphologic manifestation of ductal carcinoma in situ. Additional studies are needed to better understand the biologic nature and clinical significance of these lesions.

Lesions characterized by the presence of columnar epithelial cells lining the terminal duct lobular units (TDLUs) of the breast have long been recognized by pathologists and have been described under a wide variety of names.[1–21] In the premammographic era, columnar cell lesions were identified as incidental microscopic findings in breast tissue removed because of other abnormalities and have generally received little attention. Some of these lesions feature banal columnar cells that are in a single layer or show stratification and tufting but do not have cytologic atypia or complex architectural patterns (columnar cell change or columnar cell hyperplasia). In other lesions, the lining cells exhibit low-grade, monomorphic-type cytologic atypia and were included among lesions originally categorized by Azzopardi[4] as "clinging carcinoma" (monomorphic type). Such lesions

are now categorized as "flat epithelial atypia" (FEA).[22] Recently, there has been renewed interest in these lesions because they are being encountered with increasing frequency in breast biopsies performed because of the presence of mammographic microcalcifications.[12,13]

The purpose of this article is to review the diagnostic features, differential diagnosis, and clinical significance of FEA of the breast.

GROSS FEATURES

FEA and columnar cell lesions in general cannot be recognized grossly. As mentioned previously, the manner in which FEA is most often encountered is in biopsies performed for mammographic microcalcifications.

Key Features
FLAT EPITHELIAL ATYPIA

- Enlarged TDLUs with variably dilated acini (acini tend to be rounded in contour); involved TDLUs are often more basophilic (bluer) than normal TDLUs

- One to several layers of cuboidal to columnar epithelial cells with low-grade cytologic atypia (may be subtle); complex architectural patterns are not present

- Cuboidal to columnar cells may resemble those of tubular carcinoma

- Apical snouts are often present (may be exaggerated); intraluminal secretions may be present and prominent

- Calcifications are often present (may be psammomatous)

Department of Pathology, Beth Israel Deaconess Medical Center, Harvard Medical School, 330 Brookline Avenue, Boston, MA 02215, USA
E-mail address: lcollins@bidmc.harvard.edu

Surgical Pathology 2 (2009) 263–272
doi:10.1016/j.path.2009.02.004

MICROSCOPIC FEATURES

At scanning magnification, the TDLUs of FEA typically have a more basophilic appearance than normal TDLUs because of the increased nuclear-to-cytoplasmic ratio of the cells. The acini within the TDLUs are variably dilated, often with a very rounded contour (**Fig. 1**A). The cuboidal to columnar epithelial cells lining the acini of FEA show low-grade cytologic atypia characterized by the presence of relatively monomorphic, round to ovoid nuclei that resemble those seen in the cells of low-grade ductal carcinoma in situ (DCIS; see **Fig. 1**B). These nuclei are not regularly oriented perpendicular to the basement membrane and show an increase in the nuclear-to-cytoplasmic ratio (see **Fig. 1**C). Cellular and nuclear stratification is seen in some cases. The

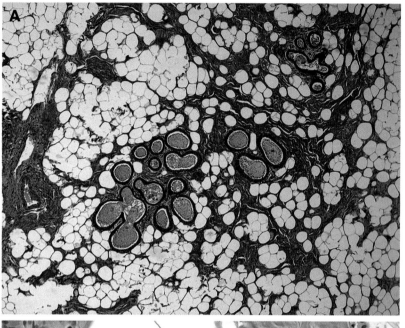

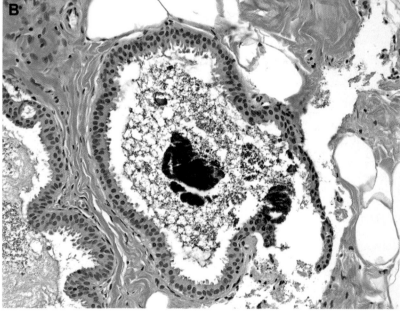

Fig. 1. (*A*) Scanning magnification of FEA showing variably dilated acini within an enlarged TDLU. At this power, the cells lining the acini appear more basophilic than is typical for microcysts, prompting a higher-power examination. (*B*) At higher power, the cuboidal nature of the cells lining the acini of FEA is evident. Some cells feature apical cytoplasmic blebs (snouts). Note also the presence of flocculent secretions and calcification.

Fig. 1. (*C*) At high power magnification, the low-grade, monomorphic cytologic atypia of FEA is readily apparent. The nuclei are rounded with variably prominent nucleoli. The cells have an increased nuclear-to-cytoplasmic ratio and are not regularly oriented with respect to the basement membrane.

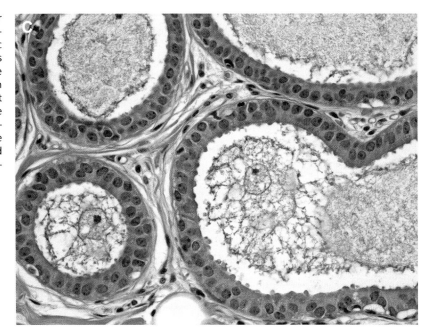

nuclear chromatin may be evenly dispersed or slightly marginated, and nucleoli are variably prominent. Mitotic figures may be seen but are uncommon. In some cases, apical cytoplasmic snouts or blebs may be prominent, and the cells cytologically may resemble those making up the tubules of tubular carcinoma (**Fig. 2**). In a minority of cases of FEA, the nuclei retain a more oval shape and orientation perpendicular to the basement membrane; however, in contrast to the relatively slender, bland nuclei of columnar cell change and columnar cell hyperplasia (see later discussion), the chromatin in these nuclei may show clumping and margination, the nucleoli are variably prominent, and the nuclear-to-cytoplasmic ratio of the cells is markedly increased. The cells of these FEA lesions are reminiscent of those seen in colonic adenomas.

Fig. 2. In this example of FEA, the cells have prominent apical cytoplasmic blebs and cytologically resemble the cells of tubular carcinoma (which was present elsewhere in this particular case). Note the coexistence of atypical lobular hyperplasia in the lower half of the image. Although not depicted in this image, this case demonstrated the "Rosen triad."

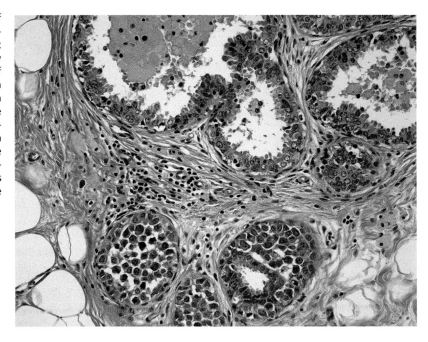

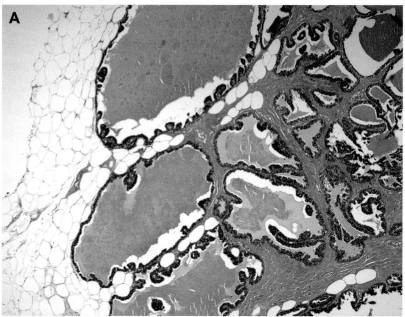

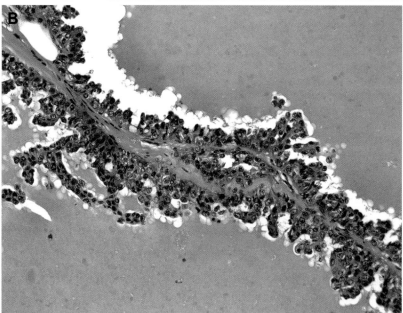

Fig. 3. Cystic hypersecretory hyperplasia (CHH). (*A*) At low-power examination, numerous cystically dilated spaces are present. The dilated spaces contain the very characteristic colloid-like secretion of CHH. Many of the spaces have a flat lining epithelium. (*B*) At high-power examination, crowding of the epithelial cells, micropapillary formations, and moderate cytologic atypia are noted in this example of CHH with atypia.

The epithelial cells in FEA lesions may form small mounds or tufts; however, complex architectural patterns, such as well-developed micropapillations, rigid cellular bridges, bars and arcades, and sieve-like fenestrations with cellular polarization within the micropapillations and arcades or around the fenestrations, are absent. Thus, "flat" is a relative term denoting the absence of complex architectural patterns. Exaggerated apical cytoplasmic snouts and abundant flocculent intraluminal secretions are often present in FEA (see **Fig. 1**B), and some of the cells composing such lesions may have a hobnail appearance. This lesion frequently shows intraluminal calcifications, which in some instances may have the configuration of psammoma bodies. A variable lymphocytic infiltrate may be present in the stroma surrounding spaces involved by FEA.

Note that high-grade cytologic atypia with marked nuclear pleomorphism of the type seen in high-grade DCIS is not a feature of lesions included in the category of FEA.[22] The presence of high-grade nuclear features warrants the designation of high-grade DCIS, even if the atypical cells compose only a single cell layer.[23] In general, such lesions are rarely seen in the absence of high-grade DCIS exhibiting other architectural patterns.

IMMUNOPHENOTYPE

Most of the cells that make up FEA and columnar cell lesions without atypia exhibit expression of cytokeratin 19[24,25] and consistently lack expression of high molecular weight cytokeratins (HMW-CK; eg, with 34βE-12 and CK5 or CK5/6).[25-28] The practical implication of this latter observation is that absence of HMW-CK expression cannot be used as an objective marker of atypia in columnar cell lesions, as has been done with other atypical intraductal proliferations (such as atypical ductal hyperplasia [ADH] and DCIS, which lack or show markedly reduced HMW-CK expression) in the distinction from usual ductal hyperplasias (which typically show a mosaic pattern of HMW-CK expression).[26,27,29]

FEA and columnar cell lesions without atypia characteristically exhibit intense nuclear expression of estrogen receptor[7,15,25,30-33] and progesterone receptor[15,24,25] in most of the cells. With regard to cell cycle and proliferation markers, the cells of FEA, even those columnar cell lesions without atypia, appear to have a higher proliferation rate and less apoptosis than normal TDLUs when evaluated for cyclin D1, Ki-67, and bcl-2.[15,24,30]

DIFFERENTIAL DIAGNOSIS

Various entities enter the differential diagnosis for FEA. First, the lesion needs to be distinguished from microcysts, which FEA resembles on low-power examination. High-power examination of dilated TDLUs is required to appreciate the subtle cytologic atypia that is present in FEA[14] but absent in microcysts, which are characterized by an attenuated cuboidal epithelium.

FEA must also be distinguished from benign apocrine lesions such as apocrine metaplasia and apocrine hyperplasia. Although the cells of FEA and apocrine lesions may feature apical cytoplasmic snouts, the cells of apocrine lesions possess more abundant, granular, eosinophilic cytoplasm than those of FEA. In addition, the nuclei of apocrine lesions tend to be round and have a single prominent nucleolus. Furthermore, whereas hobnail-type cells and highly

---

△△ **Differential Diagnosis**
FLAT EPITHELIAL ATYPIA

- Microcysts

  ○ High-power examination of dilated TDLUs reveals subtle cytologic atypia of the cuboidal epithelium present in FEA whereas microcysts are characterized by an attenuated epithelium

- Apocrine cysts

  ○ Possess more abundant, granular, eosinophilic cytoplasm than those of FEA

  ○ Nuclei tend to be round and have a single prominent nucleolus

  ○ Hobnail-type cells and highly exaggerated apical snouting seen in some examples of FEA are not seen in apocrine cysts

  ○ In contrast to FEA, apocrine epithelial cells characteristically lack expression of estrogen receptor and bcl2

- Columnar cell lesions without atypia

  ○ Columnar cell change and columnar cell hyperplasia lack the low-grade cytologic atypia characteristic of FEA

  ○ Acini more irregular in conformation in contrast to the more rounded acini seen in FEA

- Cystic hypersecretory hyperplasia (CHH)/pregnancy-like hyperplasia

  ○ Pregnancy-like hyperplasia characterized by dilated TDLUs lined by epithelial cells that often show cytoplasmic blebs that differ from those in FEA in that they are often enlarged with abundant, vacuolated cytoplasm

  ○ CHH characterized by dilated TDLUs lined by flattened epithelial cells, but acini contain characteristic colloid-like secretion to help distinguish the two entities

- Atypical ductal hyperplasia (ADH)

- Low-grade DCIS

  ○ Architectural atypia in the form of bridges and arcades is present in ADH and low-grade DCIS

exaggerated apical snouting are seen in some examples of FEA, they are not seen in apocrine lesions. Finally, in contrast to the cells of FEA, which typically show strong expression of estrogen receptor and bcl2, apocrine epithelial cells characteristically lack expression of both these proteins.[30]

Pregnancy-like hyperplasia and cystic hypersecretory hyperplasia (CHH) may also enter into the differential diagnosis.[34] The former is characterized by dilated TDLUs lined by epithelial cells that often show cytoplasmic blebs. The epithelial cells, however, differ from those in FEA in that they are often enlarged with abundant, vacuolated cytoplasm. CHH is also characterized by dilated TDLUs lined by flattened epithelial cells (sometimes with cytologic atypia), but the acini contain a very characteristic colloid-like secretion that helps in the distinction of these two entities (**Fig. 3**).[34]

Columnar cell change and columnar cell hyperplasia are recognized by their columnar cells and ovoid nuclei without prominent nucleoli, whereas in FEA, the cells tend to be more cuboidal and the nuclei are rounded with or without nucleoli as described earlier. Both columnar cell change and columnar cell hyperplasia are characterized by variably dilated acini within the TDLU, but in contrast to the more rounded acini seen in FEA, the acini seen in the columnar cell lesions without atypia tend to be more irregular in conformation (**Fig. 4**).

From a practical perspective, it is more important to distinguish columnar cell lesions without atypia from FEA than it is to distinguish columnar cell change and columnar cell hyperplasia from each other. The ability of pathologists to reproducibly distinguish columnar cell lesions without atypia (ie, columnar cell change and columnar cell hyperplasia) from FEA has been addressed in several recent studies. Reproducibility ranges from fair to excellent in these studies, with excellent interobserver agreement being reported when standardized diagnostic criteria are used.[35–37]

When FEA becomes more proliferative and begins to show architectural atypia in the form of bridges and arcades, the differential diagnostic considerations include ADH and low-grade DCIS. Lesions with low-grade cytologic atypia and sufficient architectural atypia to be classified as ADH or DCIS should be diagnosed as such.[9,38–40] Lesions that architecturally fall short of the histologic criteria for ADH or DCIS should be classified as FEA. Flat lesions without architectural atypia but in which there is high-grade cytologic atypia should be categorized as high-grade DCIS and not FEA, as discussed earlier.[41]

DIAGNOSIS

The appropriate pathology work-up and clinical management of patients whose biopsy specimens show FEA are evolving as information regarding this lesion accumulates.

CORE NEEDLE BIOPSY

Recent data have suggested that when FEA is encountered in a core needle biopsy specimen, subsequent excision shows a more advanced lesion in about one fourth to one third of cases, which is sufficiently frequent to recommend excision as a matter of routine in such cases.[42–47] In contrast, the limited available data suggest that additional pathology work-up and excision are not required when columnar cell lesions without atypia are encountered in a core needle biopsy specimen.[42,43]

EXCISIONAL BIOPSY

The presence of FEA in an excisional biopsy specimen should prompt a careful search for areas with diagnostic features of ADH or DCIS by obtaining additional levels from the block or blocks containing the lesion and by submitting the remainder of the tissue for histologic examination. Many studies have documented the presence of coexistant worse lesions in the presence of FEA (and even columnar cell lesions without atypia).[7,10–13,46,48–50] The "Rosen triad" refers to the coexistence of columnar cell lesions (with or without atypia) with lobular neoplasia and tubular carcinoma (see **Fig. 2**).[10,51,52] In addition, it has been demonstrated that FEA is more commonly associated with DCIS of low nuclear grade and micropapillary architectural pattern and with an absence of stromal desmoplasia and stromal inflammation (features more commonly associated with high-grade DCIS).[53] These observations taken together with emerging information on genetic alterations (see later discussion) in FEA lend credence to the hypothesis that FEA is part of the spectrum of lesions along the low-grade neoplasia pathway.[54,55]

It is recommended that when a proliferation fulfilling the diagnostic criteria for ADH or DCIS is found to arise in a background of FEA, the patient should be managed as one would manage ADH or DCIS in any other setting. Two issues remain to be resolved, however, when FEA is found to coexist with diagnostic areas of DCIS, particularly in cases in which the cytologic features of the cells of the FEA are identical to those of the cells of the diagnostic areas of DCIS. The first issue is whether the FEA should be taken into consideration in

Fig. 4. Columnar cell change. (*A*) Scanning magnification of columnar cell change demonstrating an enlarged TDLU with variably dilated acini (some with a more irregular contour). Microcalcifications are present. More normal-sized acini are present in the lower right of the image. (*B*) High-power image illustrating the columnar nature of the cells lining one of the cystically dilated acini. The nuclei are oval and oriented regularly with respect to the basement membrane.

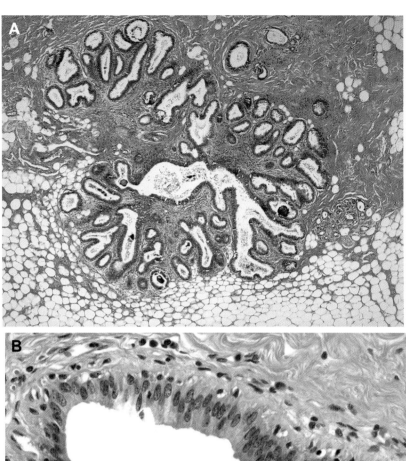

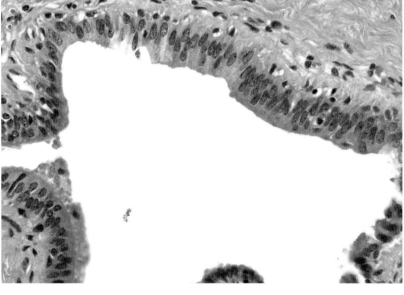

determining the size or extent of the DCIS lesion; the second is whether the presence of FEA at the excision margins is sufficient to consider the margins "positive," requiring further surgical resection. Given that the available clinical data, albeit limited, suggest that FEA is associated with a very low risk of recurrence or progression to invasive carcinoma (see later discussion), it should probably not be taken into consideration when

determining the size of a coexistent DCIS lesion or when evaluating the status of the margins of excision, even when the lesion comprises cells that are cytologically similar to those in the diagnostic areas of DCIS.[48,52]

Another increasingly common problem is the management of patients whose breast biopsy tissue, after thorough examination, shows FEA without diagnostic areas of ADH or DCIS. It has been argued that despite the fact that this lesion may well be neoplastic and even composed of cells that are identical to those seen in some forms of DCIS or even tubular carcinoma, the few available clinical follow-up studies of FEA suggest that it is associated with a risk of subsequent breast cancer that is considerably lower than that seen with fully developed forms of low-grade DCIS (see later discussion).[48] Therefore, managing patients who have such lesions as if they had DCIS would result in overtreatment of many patients.

PROGNOSIS

It is difficult to assess the clinical significance of FEA because of variations in the terminology used in the literature to describe this lesion and the limited number of cases that have been studied in a formal manner. Nonetheless, several observational studies have clearly shown that the lesion now recognized as FEA commonly coexists with well-developed examples of ADH, low-grade DCIS, and tubular carcinoma and that the cells of the FEA share cytologic and immunophenotypic features with the cells of these other lesions.[6,7,9–14,23,49,56] A number of investigators have also noted an association between FEA and lobular neoplasia (lobular carcinoma in situ and atypical lobular hyperplasia).[10,50–52,56]

Given these observations and in conjunction with studies that have reported similar genetic alterations in FEA as found in adjacent foci of DCIS and invasive carcinoma (most frequently involving 11q and 16q),[14,25,57] it is reasonable to conclude that FEA is a neoplastic proliferation that may well represent a precursor to, or the earliest morphologic manifestation of, low-grade DCIS and a precursor to invasive carcinoma, particularly tubular carcinoma.[54,55] The clinical significance of these observations, however, can be determined only from follow-up studies.

To date, few follow-up studies have directly addressed the clinical significance of lesions currently categorized as FEA. In a review of over 9000 breast biopsy specimens that were initially considered benign, Eusebi and colleagues[23] retrospectively identified 25 patients who had so-called "clinging carcinoma" of the flat, monomorphic (low nuclear grade) type (FEA). Only one of these patients (4%) developed a "local recurrence" of a histologically identical lesion after an average follow-up period of 19.2 years, without progression to DCIS or invasive carcinoma. In another study that examined 59 patients who had clinging carcinoma of the low nuclear grade type (FEA),[58] there were no local recurrences (median follow-up, 5.4 years). Recently, de Mascarel and colleagues[46]

Pitfalls
FLAT EPITHELIAL ATYPIA

! Cases with FEA may harbor other worse lesions, such as

  ! ADH

  ! Low-grade DCIS

  ! Tubular carcinoma

  ! Lobular neoplasia (lobular carcinoma in situ or atypical lobular hyperplasia)

reported that none of 84 patients who had FEA as an isolated lesion on excision progressed to a worse lesion in 10 years of follow-up. Most recently, Boulos and colleagues[48] reported that the presence of columnar cell lesions (with and without atypia) were associated with only a mild increase in subsequent breast cancer risk (relative risk, 1.47) and that there was no significant difference in risk among the three categories of columnar cell lesions (ie, columnar cell change, columnar cell hyperplasia, and FEA), although numbers were small in the case-control portion of that study.

Thus, the limited data available suggest that among patients who have FEA, the likelihood of progression to invasive breast cancer is exceedingly low.

Additional clinical follow-up studies are needed to better understand the relationship between FEA and the risk of subsequent breast cancer.

SUMMARY

FEA is encountered with increasing frequency in breast biopsies performed because of mammographic microcalcifications. Emerging data suggest that FEA is a neoplastic, clonal proliferation that may represent a precursor to or the earliest form of low-grade DCIS. Nonetheless, the limited available clinical follow-up data suggest that the risk of progression of this lesion to invasive cancer appears to be extraordinarily low, supporting the notion that categorizing FEA as clinging carcinoma and managing such lesions as if they were fully developed DCIS would result in overtreatment of many patients. For the practicing pathologist, the identification of FEA in a breast biopsy specimen should serve as a red flag for the possible presence of coexisting ADH, DCIS, lobular neoplasia, and invasive carcinoma (particularly tubular carcinoma).

REFERENCES

1. Page DL, Anderson TJ. Diagnostic histopathology of the breast. Edinburgh (Scotland): Churchill Livingstone; 1987.
2. Trojani M. Atlas en couleurs d'histopathologie mammaire. Paris: Maloine; 1988 [in French].
3. Foote FW Jr, Stewart FW. Comparative studies of cancerous vs. non-cancerous breasts. Basic morphological characteristics. Ann Surg 1945;121:6–53.
4. Azzopardi JG. Problems in breast pathology. Philadelphia: WB Saunders; 1979.
5. Gallager HS. Sources of uncertainty in interpretation of breast biopsies. Breast 1976;2:12–5.
6. Wellings SR, Jensen HM, Marcum RG. An atlas of subgross pathology of the human breast with special reference to possible precancerous lesions. J Natl Cancer Inst 1975;55(2):231–73.
7. Oyama T, Iijima K, Takei H, et al. Atypical cystic lobule of the breast: an early stage of low-grade ductal carcinoma in-situ. Breast Cancer 2000;7(4):326–31.
8. Tsuchiya S. Atypical ductal hyperplasia, atypical lobular hyperplasia, and interpretation of a new borderline lesion. Jpn J Cancer Clin 1998;44:548–55.
9. Rosen PP. Rosen's breast pathology. 2nd edition. Philadelphia: Lippincott-Raven; 2001.
10. Rosen PP. Columnar cell hyperplasia is associated with lobular carcinoma in situ and tubular carcinoma. Am J Surg Pathol 1999;23(12):1561.
11. Goldstein NS, O'Malley BA. Cancerization of small ectatic ducts of the breast by ductal carcinoma in situ cells with apocrine snouts: a lesion associated with tubular carcinoma. Am J Clin Pathol 1997;107(5):561–6.
12. Page DL, Kasami M, Jensen RA. Hypersecretory hyperplasia with atypia in breast biopsies. What is the proper level of clinical concern? Pathol Case Reviews 1996;1:36–40.
13. Fraser JL, Raza S, Chorny K, et al. Columnar alteration with prominent apical snouts and secretions: a spectrum of changes frequently present in breast biopsies performed for microcalcifications. Am J Surg Pathol 1998;22(12):1521–7.
14. Moinfar F, Man YG, Bratthauer GL, et al. Genetic abnormalities in mammary ductal intraepithelial neoplasia-flat type ("clinging ductal carcinoma in situ"): a simulator of normal mammary epithelium. Cancer 2000;88(9):2072–81.
15. Lee S, Mohsin SK, Mao S, et al. Hormones, receptors, and growth in hyperplastic enlarged lobular units: early potential precursors of breast cancer. Breast Cancer Res 2006;8(1):R6.
16. McLaren BK, Gobbi H, Schuyler PA, et al. Immunohistochemical expression of estrogen receptor in enlarged lobular units with columnar alteration in benign breast biopsies: a nested case-control study. Am J Surg Pathol 2005;29(1):105–8.
17. Mohsin SK, Allred DC, Osborne CK, et al. Morphologic and immunophenotypic markers as surrogate endpoints of tamoxifen effect for prevention of breast cancer. Breast Cancer Res Treat 2005; 94(3):205–11.
18. Arpino G, Laucirica R, Elledge RM. Premalignant and in situ breast disease: biology and clinical implications. Ann Intern Med 2005;143(6):446–57.
19. Schnitt SJ. The diagnosis and management of pre-invasive breast disease: flat epithelial atypia—classification, pathologic features and clinical significance. Breast Cancer Res 2003;5(5):263–8.
20. Schnitt SJ. Columnar cell lesions of the breast: pathologic features and clinical significance. Current Diag Pathol 2004;10:193–203.
21. Nasser SM. Columnar cell lesions: current classification and controversies. Semin Diagn Pathol 2004; 21(1):18–24.
22. Tavassoli FA, Hoefler H, Rosai J, et al. Intraductal proliferative lesions. In: Tavassoli FA, Devilee P. editors. Pathology and genetics: tumours of the breast and female genital organs. Lyon (France): IARC Press; 2003. p. 63–73.
23. Eusebi V, Feudale E, Foschini MP, et al. Long-term follow-up of in situ carcinoma of the breast. Semin Diagn Pathol 1994;11(3):223–35.
24. Oyama T, Maluf H, Koerner F. Atypical cystic lobules: an early stage in the formation of low-grade ductal carcinoma in situ. Virchows Arch 1999; 435(4):413–21.
25. Simpson PT, Gale T, Reis-Filho JS, et al. Columnar cell lesions of the breast: the missing link in breast cancer progression?: a morphological and molecular analysis. Am J Surg Pathol 2005;29(6):734–46.
26. Otterbach F, Bankfalvi A, Bergner S, et al. Cytokeratin 5/6 immunohistochemistry assists the differential diagnosis of atypical proliferations of the breast. Histopathology 2000;37(3):232–40.
27. Carlo V, Fraser J, Pliss N, et al. Can absence of high molecular weight cytokeratin expression be used as a marker of atypia in columnar cell lesions of the breast? Mod Pathol 2003;16:24A.
28. Raju U, Ornsby A, Ma C, et al. Columnar cell changes in breast: when are they atypical? An immunohistochemical study of cytokeratin 5/6 (CK5/6) and hormone receptor expression. Lab Invest 2004;17(Suppl 1):46A.
29. Moinfar F, Man YG, Lininger RA, et al. Use of keratin 35betaE12 as an adjunct in the diagnosis of mammary intraepithelial neoplasia-ductal type—benign and malignant intraductal proliferations. Am J Surg Pathol 1999;23(9):1048–58.
30. Fraser JL, Roya S, Chorny K, et al. Immunophenotype of columnar alteration with prominent apical snouts and secretions (CAPSS). Lab Invest 2000; 80:21A.

31. Allred DC, Mohsin SK, Fuqua SA. Histological and biological evolution of human premalignant breast disease. Endocr Relat Cancer 2001;8(1):47–61.

32. Dabbs DJ, Kessinger RL, McManus K, et al. Biology of columnar cell lesions in core biopsies of the breast. Mod Pathol 2003;16:26A.

33. Tremblay G, Deschenes J, Alpert L, et al. Overexpression of estrogen receptors in columnar cell change and in unfolding breast lobules. Breast J 2005;11(5):326–32.

34. Feeley L, Quinn CM. Columnar cell lesions of the breast. Histopathology 2008;52(1):11–9.

35. Mohsin S, Badve S, Bose S, et al. Assessment of variability in diagnosing "atypia" in columnar cell lesions (CCL) of the breast. Lab Invest 2005; 85(Suppl 1):44A.

36. O'Malley FP, Mohsin SK, Badve S, et al. Interobserver reproducibility in the diagnosis of flat epithelial atypia of the breast. Mod Pathol 2006;19(2):172–9.

37. Tan PH, Ho BC, Selvarajan S, et al. Pathological diagnosis of columnar cell lesions of the breast: are there issues of reproducibility? J Clin Pathol 2005;58(7):705–9.

38. Dupont WD, Page DL. Risk factors for breast cancer in women with proliferative breast disease. N Engl J Med 1985;312(3):146–51.

39. Page DL, Dupont WD, Rogers LW, et al. Atypical hyperplastic lesions of the female breast. A long-term follow-up study. Cancer 1985;55(11):2698–708.

40. Page DL, Rogers LW. Combined histologic and cytologic criteria for the diagnosis of mammary atypical ductal hyperplasia. Hum Pathol 1992;23(10): 1095–7.

41. Schnitt SJ, Vincent-Salomon A. Columnar cell lesions of the breast. Adv Anat Pathol 2003;10(3): 113–24.

42. Brogi E, Tan LK. Findings at excisional biopsy (EBX) performed after identification of columnar cell change (CCC) of ductal epithelium in breast core biopsy (CBX). [Meeting abstract]. Mod Pathol 2002;15(1):29A–30A.

43. Harigopal M, Yao DX, Hoda SA, et al. Columnar cell alteration diagnosed on mammotome core biopsy for indeterminate microcalcifications: results of subsequent mammograms and surgical excision. Mod Pathol 2002;15:36A.

44. Nasser S, Fan MJ. Does atypical columnar cell hyperplasia on breast core biopsy warrant follow-up excision? Mod Pathol 2003;16:42A.

45. Kunju LP, Kleer CG. Significance of flat epithelial atypia on mammotome core needle biopsy: should it be excised? Hum Pathol 2007;38(1):35–41.

46. de Mascarel I, MacGrogan G, Mathoulin-Pelissier S, et al. Epithelial atypia in biopsies performed for microcalcifications. Practical considerations about 2,833 serially sectioned surgical biopsies with a long follow-up. Virchows Arch 2007;451(1):1–10.

47. Martel M, Barron-Rodriguez P, Tolgay Ocal I, et al. Flat DIN 1 (flat epithelial atypia) on core needle biopsy: 63 cases identified retrospectively among 1,751 core biopsies performed over an 8-year period (1992–1999). Virchows Arch 2007;451(5): 883–91.

48. Boulos FI, Dupont WD, Simpson JF, et al. Histologic associations and long-term cancer risk in columnar cell lesions of the breast: a retrospective cohort and a nested case-control study. Cancer 2008; 113(9):2415–21.

49. Weidner N. Malignant breast lesions that may mimic benign tumors. Semin Diagn Pathol 1995;12(1): 2–13.

50. Brogi E, Oyama T, Koerner FC. Atypical cystic lobules in patients with lobular neoplasia. Int J Surg Pathol 2001;9(3):201–6.

51. Brandt SM, Young GQ, Hoda SA. The "Rosen triad": tubular carcinoma, lobular carcinoma in situ, and columnar cell lesions. Adv Anat Pathol 2008;15(3): 140–6.

52. Leibl S, Regitnig P, Moinfar F. Flat epithelial atypia (DIN 1a, atypical columnar change): an underdiagnosed entity very frequently coexisting with lobular neoplasia. Histopathology 2007;50(7):859–65.

53. Collins LC, Achacoso NA, Nekhlyudov L, et al. Clinical and pathologic features of ductal carcinoma in situ associated with the presence of flat epithelial atypia: an analysis of 543 patients. Mod Pathol 2007;20(11):1149–55.

54. Abdel-Fatah TM, Powe DG, Hodi Z, et al. High frequency of coexistence of columnar cell lesions, lobular neoplasia, and low grade ductal carcinoma in situ with invasive tubular carcinoma and invasive lobular carcinoma. Am J Surg Pathol 2007;31(3): 417–26.

55. Turashvili G, McKinney S, Martin L, et al. Columnar cell lesions, mammographic density and breast cancer risk. Breast Cancer Res Treat 2008.

56. Sahoo S, Recant WM. Triad of columnar cell alteration, lobular carcinoma in situ, and tubular carcinoma of the breast. Breast J 2005;11(2):140–2.

57. Dabbs DJ, Carter G, Fudge M, et al. Molecular alterations in columnar cell lesions of the breast. Mod Pathol 2006;19(3):344–9.

58. Bijker N, Peterse JL, Duchateau L, et al. Risk factors for recurrence and metastasis after breast-conserving therapy for ductal carcinoma-in-situ: analysis of European Organization for Research and Treatment of Cancer Trial 10853. J Clin Oncol 2001;19(8):2263–71.

LOBULAR CARCINOMA IN SITU, CLASSICAL TYPE AND UNUSUAL VARIANTS

Melissa Murray, DO*, Edi Brogi, MD, PhD

KEYWORDS

- Breast • Lobular carcinoma in situ • Lobular neoplasia • Pleomorphic lobular carcinoma in situ
- Carcinoma in situ with indeterminate features • Diagnosis • Breast cancer • E-cadherin

ABSTRACT

The morphologic spectrum of lobular carcinoma in situ (LCIS) includes the classical type and unusual variants recently described. In this article we review the morphology of LCIS and highlight ways to distinguish it from its morphologic mimickers.

In the first description of lobular carcinoma in situ (LCIS) in 1941, Foote and Stewart[1] suggested that this lesion was a precursor of breast carcinoma. Subsequent studies, however, concluded that LCIS was only a risk factor, not a true precursor. Over 60 years later, multiple lines of evidence have shed new light on LCIS, reviving the hypothesis of a precursor lesion. Furthermore, recent molecular and immunophenotypic studies have shown that some solid mammary carcinomas in situ with necrosis and calcifications, previously classified as ductal carcinoma in situ (DCIS), show lobular differentiation. The broadened spectrum of neoplastic lobular proliferations raises new questions on the biology of the disease, and the appropriate management of its morphologic variants. In this article, we review the morphologic and immunophenotypic features of in situ proliferations showing lobular differentiation, and discuss some issues related to their clinical management.

LOBULAR CARCINOMA IN SITU, CLASSICAL TYPE

Lobular carcinoma in situ, classical type (C-LCIS) usually constitutes an incidental microscopic finding and its incidence in the general population remains unknown. The mean age at diagnosis ranges between 44–54 years. Some studies have suggested that the incidence of C-LCIS in postmenopausal women has increased, but this may just reflect an increase in the radiologic detection of LCIS-associated lesions, or increased ability of pathologists to recognize this lesion.[2]

GROSS FEATURES

C-LCIS has no specific mammographic correlate.[3] Mammographic calcifications are often the indication for a breast biopsy yielding C-LCIS, but they are usually associated with a nonneoplastic proliferation adjacent to C-LCIS, such as sclerosing adenosis. Rarely, C-LCIS contains minute calcifications, likely due to colonization of a preexisting calcified focus. C-LCIS is also frequently associated with flat epithelial atypia,[4] and the latter lesion typically harbors laminated calcifications. C-LCIS has no distinguishing features on gross examination.

Department of Pathology, Memorial Sloan-Kettering Cancer Center, Weill Cornell Medical College, 1275 York Avenue, New York, NY 10065, USA
* Corresponding author.
E-mail address: murraym@mskcc.org (M. Murray).

Surgical Pathology 2 (2009) 273–299
doi:10.1016/j.path.2009.02.001

Key Features
LOBULAR CARCINOMA IN SITU, CLASSICAL TYPE

1. C-LCIS is not associated with a specific mammographic or gross abnormality

2. The acini are filled and distended by a monotonous proliferation of small discohesive cells

3. Intracytoplasmic vacuoles with "targetoid inclusions" are frequent and can indent the nucleus (signet ring cell morphology)

4. Intracytoplasmic mucin can indent the nucleus (signet ring cell morphology)

5. C-LCIS extends along the basement membrane of extralobular ducts, lifting up the native luminal epithelium ("pagetoid growth")

6. A cross-section of an extralobular duct involved by C-LCIS shows "clover-leaf" appearance

7. C-LCIS lacks membranous reactivity for E-cadherin, and shows cytoplasmic positivity for 34βE12 and p120

LCIS has been traditionally considered a risk lesion. Recent evidence suggests that C-LCIS constitutes a nonobligate precursor of breast carcinoma, but its progression may be very slow. Thus, margin status of C-LCIS is not reported and radiation is not used in treatment.

MICROSCOPIC FEATURES

Lobules involved by C-LCIS are distended by a monotonous proliferation of small cells that expand the acini and obliterate their lumen. The cells typically show loss of cohesion (**Fig. 1**). As a result, each tumor cell is surrounded by irregular "empty" spaces, imparting a rarefied appearance to the involved lobules, on low-power examination. The cells have a narrow rim of pale to lightly eosinophilic cytoplasm, and a centrally located nucleus, with round-to-oval shape. The resulting morphology is often described as that of a fried egg. The nuclei are small and uniform, and show only slight membrane irregularity and fine, homogenous chromatin; nucleoli are absent or inconspicuous. Haagensen and colleagues[5] referred to LCIS cells with this morphology as type A cells (**Fig. 2**). Haagensen,[5] Azzopardi,[6] and other pathologists[7] also noted that some C-LCIS lesions consist of larger cells with more abundant cytoplasm, and enlarged nuclei with slightly irregular nuclear membranes and evident nucleoli. Cells with this

morphology are referred to as type B cells (using Haagensen's terminology[5]) or as large cells of C-LCIS (**Fig. 3**). LCIS type A and type B cells often occur in close proximity and can coexist within the same lobule (**Fig. 4**).

Mucin-filled intracytoplasmic vacuoles are a frequent and characteristic feature of C-LCIS, and can appear as targetoid inclusions. Ultrastructural studies have shown that these vacuoles consist of intracytoplasmic glandular lumina.[8] They may be quite large and indent the nucleus, resulting in signet ring cell morphology. The latter appearance, can also be secondary to intracytoplasmic accumulation of mucin, another frequent feature of C-LCIS.

Mitoses and necrosis are not typical of C-LCIS, and their identification should prompt critical re-evaluation of the lesion to rule out a special variant of LCIS.

The diagnosis of C-LCIS requires expansion of the acini of a lobule (**Fig. 5**), but no definite criteria exist regarding the extent of distention, the minimum number of acini that need to be involved, or the number of affected lobules necessary for the diagnosis. According to Page,[9] the diagnosis of C-LCIS requires distension of at least 50% of the acini of one lobule, whereas Rosen[10] requires involvement of at least 75%. Less-developed lesions are classified as atypical lobular hyperplasia (ALH) (section on ALH follows). Because the distinction between C-LCIS and ALH is quantitative rather than qualitative, interobserver and even intraobserver variability are not infrequent.

As the name implies, C-LCIS is a lobulocentric lesion, but it often extends to involve extralobular ducts, as Foote and Stewart noted in their seminal report.[1] C-LCIS cells grow along the basement membrane of the duct and undermine the native epithelium, lifting it up toward the lumen. Ductal extension of C-LCIS can consist of single cells, small nests, or very large sheets. The growth of LCIS in extralobular ducts is referred to as "pagetoid" due to its resemblance to the intraepidermal spread of adenocarcinoma in Paget's disease of the nipple. A flattened layer of attenuated ductal cells typically persists between LCIS and the duct lumen (**Fig. 6**). The so-called "cloverleaf" configuration of a duct cross-section is due to focal expansion of the wall by C-LCIS, resulting in regular bulbous protrusions into the periductal stroma (**Fig. 7**).

In C-LCIS, the myoepithelium lining ducts and lobules persist, and can often be hyperplastic. The cytoplasm of myoepithelial cells admixed with C-LCIS is inconspicuous, but the myoepithelial nuclei are easily identified among the neoplastic cells due to their crescentic shape and dense

Fig. 1. Lobular carcinoma in situ, classical type (C-LCIS). (*A*) The cells of C-LCIS show loss of cohesion (100×). (*B*) The tumor cells are surrounded by a narrow rim of eosinophilic cytoplasm and irregular empty spaces (400×).

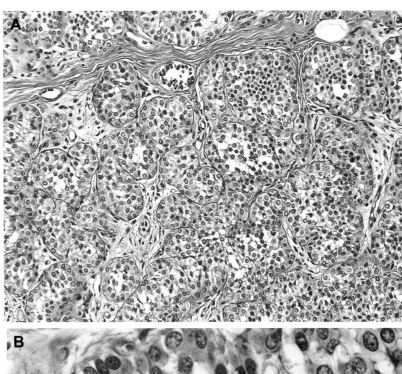

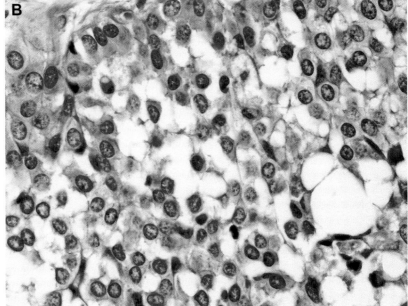

chromatin. Focal matrix deposition is often present in cases of C-LCIS associated with myoepithelial hyperplasia.

LOBULAR CARCINOMA IN SITU IN THE ATROPHIC BREAST

In postmenopausal women, the terminal duct lobular units of the breast undergo physiologic involution and ultimately disappear. In this setting, the degree of lobular expansion diagnostic of LCIS is not as obvious as in younger women. Because lobules are sparse and have only a few small acini, C-LCIS can manifest itself as just a single layer of tumor cells undermining the native epithelium of extralobular ducts. Thus, C-LCIS occurring in the breasts of older women can be easily overlooked. A similar subtle pattern

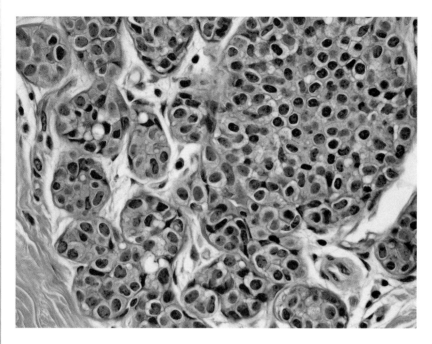

Fig. 2. Lobular carcinoma in situ, classical type with type A cells. A few cells show intracytoplasmic vacuoles and signet ring cell morphology (400×).

of C-LCIS can sometimes be observed in irradiated breast tissue.

DIFFERENTIAL DIAGNOSIS

The differential diagnosis of C-LCIS consists of two types of lesions: (1) Lesions that mimic C-LCIS and (2) C-LCIS in a nonneoplastic proliferation, mimicking a more severe lesion.

Lesions that Mimic Lobular Carcinoma In Situ, Classical Type

Ductal carcinoma in situ, low nuclear grade
DCIS with low nuclear grade and solid growth into lobules can closely mimic C-LCIS. Morphologic clues indicative of ductal differentiation include polarity of the neoplastic cells, more evident in the cells resting on the basement membrane,

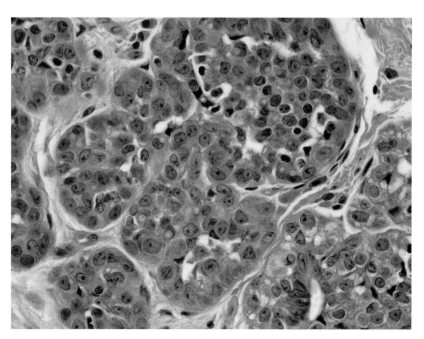

Fig. 3. Lobular carcinoma in situ, classical type (C-LCIS) with type B cells. Nucleoli are evident and nuclear membranes have more irregularities than type A cells (400×). Few intracytoplasmic vacuoles are present.

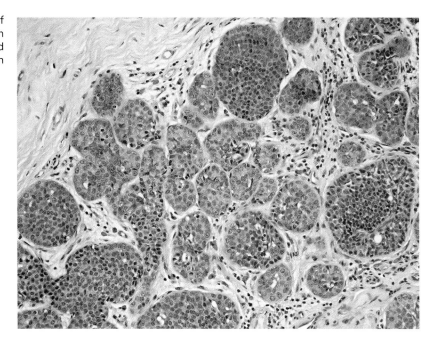

Fig. 4. Morphology of lobular carcinoma in situ, classical, type A and type B cells coexisting in the same lobule (200×).

and focal formation of microacini. DCIS cells involving a lobule show a polygonal outline with distinct cytoplasmic borders but this feature is not entirely specific. Conversely, loss of cohesion and intracytoplasmic "targetoid inclusions" favor C-LCIS. Associated pagetoid involvement of ducts is also more frequent in C-LCIS than low-grade DCIS (**Table 1**). The use of ancillary immunoperoxidase stains, namely E-cadherin (see paragraph on E-cadherin) can help to resolve problematic cases. The diagnostic differential between C-LCIS and low-grade DCIS should always be pursued, as management of these two lesions differs greatly. Coexistence of C-LCIS and DCIS in the same duct or lobule is a rare event.

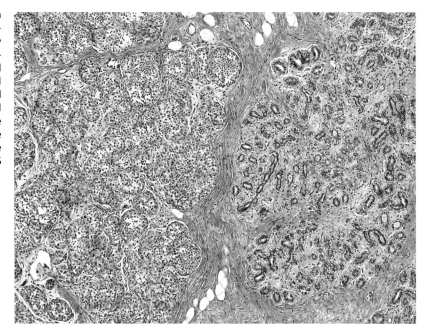

Fig. 5. Lobular carcinoma in situ, classical type (C-LCIS) expands mammary lobules. The lobules involved by C-LCIS show marked distention and overall expansion (*left*) compared with adjacent normal breast tissue (*right*). Notice the obliteration of the acinar lumina in the lobules affected by C-LCIS (100×).

△△ *Differential Diagnosis*
LOBULAR CARCINOMA IN SITU,
CLASSICAL TYPE

- Ductal carcinoma in situ, low grade

  o Cell polarity and focal microacini support ductal differentiation

  o DCIS cells show a polygonal outline and distinct cytoplasmic borders

  o In contrast to DCIS, LCIS shows discohesive cells, intracytoplasmic "targetoid inclusions," and more frequently associated pagetoid involvement of ducts

  o Use E-cadherin to resolve problematic cases

- Myoepithelial hyperplasia

  o Abundant cytoplasm and small, round, centrally located nuclei of myoepithelial cells can mimic C-LCIS

  o Hyperplastic myoepithelium in papillomas and other sclerosing lesions has regular organized distribution along the basement membrane

  o Intracytoplasmic targetoid inclusions and signet ring cell morphology support LCIS

  o Use immunoperoxidase stains for myoepithelial cells resolve problematic cases

- Special types of LCIS with type A and type B cells

  o Massive acinar expansion, central necrosis are present in S-LCIS

  o Mitoses are usually common

  o Calcifications are common.

Myoepithelial hyperplasia

In the luteal phase of the menstrual cycle, the myoepithelial cells display abundant cytoplasm and small, round, centrally located nuclei. This morphology can closely mimic that of C-LCIS, undermining normal luminal epithelium. In this setting, however, the lobules are not expanded, and the acinar lumina are patent and lined by polarized cells also showing luteal phase changes, which include enlarged nuclei with prominent nucleoli. Hyperplastic myoepithelial cells with ample cytoplasm can also be seen in papillomas, radial scars, sclerosing adenosis, and other

sclerosing lesions, but the organized distribution of the myoepithelium along the basement membrane is usually sufficient to solve the differential diagnosis. Intracytoplasmic targetoid inclusions and signet ring cell morphology support lobular differentiation. Immunoperoxidase stains for myoepithelial cells, including calponin and p63, a nuclear antigen, are helpful in problematic cases.

Clear cell change

The descriptive term "clear cell change" applies to an alteration of the epithelium of the terminal duct lobular unit characterized by clearing of the cytoplasm. No specific etiology has been reported. The cells usually have abundant cytoplasm, small dark nuclei, and no nucleoli. Clear cell change can involve an entire lobule or only part of it. It rarely associates with calcifications and usually constitutes an incidental finding.

The clear cytoplasm resembles an empty space and simulates the loss of cohesion characteristic of C-LCIS. Careful inspection, however, reveals polygonal and cohesive clear cells, with sharply defined cell membranes, and perinuclear clearing located on the intracytoplasmic side of the cell membrane. Use of immunoperoxidase stains for E-cadherin helps to sort out problematic cases.

Secretory (pregnancy-like) hyperplasia

Secretory (pregnancy-like) hyperplasia is an idiopathic change and can occur in the breast regardless of pregnancy. The affected lobules resemble those of late pregnancy and lactation, but the changes are usually focal. The acini are dilated and lined by a single layer of cuboidal-to-columnar cells with abundant delicate cytoplasm that is pale-to-clear and finely granular or vacuolated. The nuclei are typically small, round, and darkly stained. Sometimes the nuclei protrude into the gland lumen, giving the cells a hobnail appearance not a feature of C-LCIS. Secretory material is often present within the distended lumina and can contain mammographically detectable calcifications.

Tissue preservation

Poor tissue preservation may mimic C-LCIS. The cells within the lobules appear discohesive, but no real cell proliferation or lobular distension is present. On higher power examination, the cells do not display the cytologic features of C-LCIS, and show lack of nuclear and cytoplasmic detail due to poor preservation. In questionable cases,

Fig. 6. Pagetoid extension of lobular carcinoma in situ, classical type (C-LCIS) cells into a duct. C-LCIS undermines the native ductal epithelium, which is still visible as a flattened layer along the duct lumen. Buds of C-LCIS cells protruding outward from the duct wall result in a serrated pattern (400×).

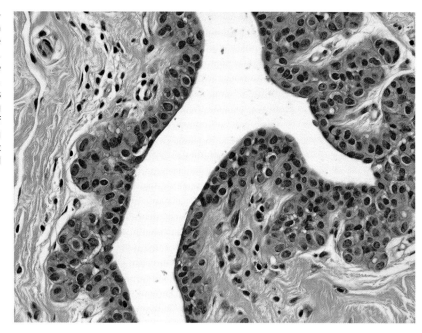

evaluation of recut sections and/or application of immunostains for E-cadherin can be helpful. In these instances, only positive immunoreactivity can be reliably interpreted, whereas a negative stain is inconclusive, as it could be secondary to antigen degradation. As a general rule, no definitive diagnosis of C-LCIS, or of any other lesion, should be rendered on poorly preserved material.

Lobular Carcinoma In Situ, Classical Type, in a Nonneoplastic Proliferation, Mimicking a More Severe Lesion

Sclerosing lesions

C-LCIS frequently involves sclerosing lesions and can closely simulate invasive carcinoma. In the evaluation of these cases, low-power examination is very helpful to appreciate the architecture of the

Fig. 7. Lobular carcinoma in situ, classical type (C-LCIS) involving a duct. Nests of C-LCIS cells located beneath the ductal epithelium protrude outward around the duct periphery resulting in a cloverleaf pattern (200×).

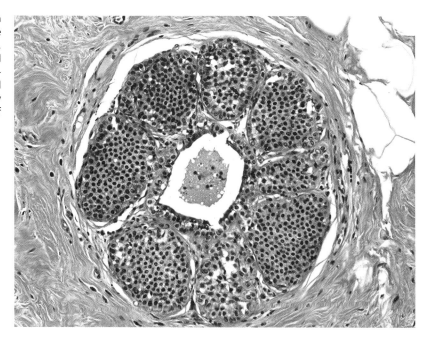

Table 1
Morphologic features of LCIS and DCIS

	C-LCIS	S-LCIS	DCIS
Cohesive growth	Absent	Absent	Present
Involvement of ducts	Pagetoid spread	Solid growth	Cribriform, solid, micropapillary
Involvement of lobules	Typical, acinar distension	Typical, massive expansion	Possible, lobular cancerization
Cell morphology	Round "fried egg"	Round-to-ovoid (plasmacytoid)	Columnar
Cytoplasm	Scant	Abundant	Variable
Nuclear pleomorphism	Absent	Absent/present	Absent/present
Nucleoli	Rare	Common	Common
Mitoses	Absent	Common	Common
Necrosis	Absent	Common	Common
Calcifications	Not typical	Frequent	Frequent
Interdigitating myoepithelium	Common	Focally present	Absent
Invasive carcinoma	Possible	Frequent	Possible

Abbreviations: C-LCIS = classical LCIS; S-LCIS = special variants of LCIS.

underlying proliferation. Sclerosing adenosis shows a characteristic swirling, lobulocentric pattern, whereas a radial scar has a zonal architecture consisting of a central, scarred nidus surrounded by hyperplastic ducts and, peripheral, large cysts. At high magnification, the compressed and elongated tubules involved by C-LCIS show an attenuated myoepithelium cells and are surrounded by a eosinophilic and refractile basement membrane. It is useful to compare these foci with adjacent areas of sclerosis uninvolved by C-LCIS. Problematic cases can usually be resolved with the aid of myoepithelial markers (**Fig. 8**).

Collagenous spherulosis

Collagenous spherulosis (CS) is a benign alteration more frequent in ducts than in lobules and often occurs in the context of a sclerosing lesion, such as a sclerosing papilloma. In CS, hyperplastic myoepithelium lays abundant extracellular matrix into acellular spherules that can be dense and eosinophilic or consist of fibrillary ground substance. The latter deposits are often translucent and can resemble empty glandular lumina. Myoepithelial cells, with flattened nuclei, encircle the spherules. The basement membrane is often visible as an eosinophilic and refractile layer interposed between the myoepithelium and spherules. LCIS may proliferate in this context and surround clear spaces of CS. On low-power examination, this pattern simulates DCIS with

low nuclear grade and cribriform architecture (**Fig. 9**). To resolve this differential diagnosis, one should start by examining the content of the round spaces. The spherules of CS are solid collections of matrix-like material surrounded by a layer of basement membrane and myoepithelium, and are usually variable in size. In contrast, the cribriform spaces of DCIS constitute neoformed lumina and thus are empty, with similar diameter, and lined by neoplastic polarized cells with columnar morphology. Degenerative changes can occur within the spherules of CS and result in collapse and focal detachment of the peripheral basement membrane from the surrounding myoepithelium. In these cases, a dense refractile bar of basement membrane forms a cord cutting across the pseudolumen, a morphologic finding that confirms the presence of CS. Attention to these features is usually sufficient to diagnose C-LCIS involving CS without resorting to the use of E-cadherin or myoepithelial markers.

LCIS involving CS usually has classic morphology, but unusual cytology may be seen focally.

Usual ductal hyperplasia

Rarely, C-LCIS involving a focus of usual ductal hyperplasia (UDH) simulates atypical ductal hyperplasia (ADH) or even low-grade DCIS. UDH can fill the lumen of a duct partially involved by C-LCIS,

Fig. 8. Lobular carcinoma in situ, classical type involving sclerosing adenosis mimics invasive carcinoma. (*A*) The compressed and elongated tubules of sclerosing adenosis are outlined by a thick eosinophilic basement membrane (200×). (*B*) Immunohistochemical stain for calponin highlights the myoepithelial cells of the sclerosed tubules (400×).

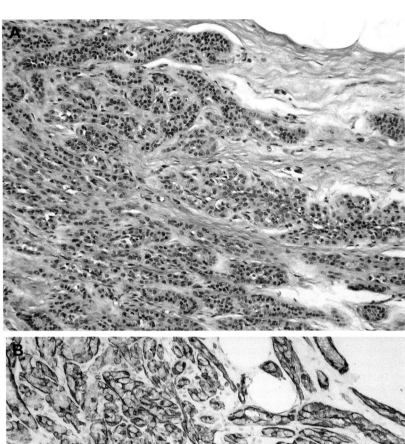

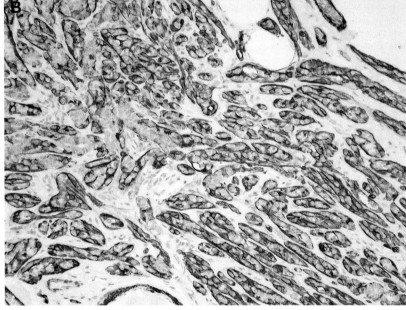

raising the differential diagnosis of solid DCIS. The residual lumen is embedded in a monotonous neoplastic proliferation, and simulates a cribriform space. Closer examination reveals that the open lumen is lined by a reduced layer of cells with dense nuclei, in contrast to the "fried egg" morphology and open chromatin of the surrounding C-LCIS.

On the other hand, foci of C-LCIS involving UDH may be underrecognized. In these cases, C-LCIS appears as a second cell population consisting of paler cells with distinct cell borders and "fried egg" morphology, scattered throughout the proliferation of UDH. Neither acinar cells nor myoepithelial cells typically have intracytoplasmic vacuoles characteristic of C-LCIS (**Fig. 10**).

In difficult cases, the use of E-cadherin will help resolve the differential diagnosis.

PROGNOSIS

In their seminal report, Foote and Stewart[1] hypothesized that LCIS was a precursor of

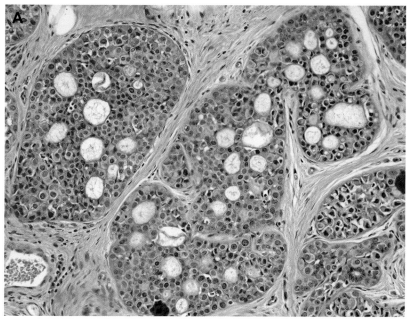

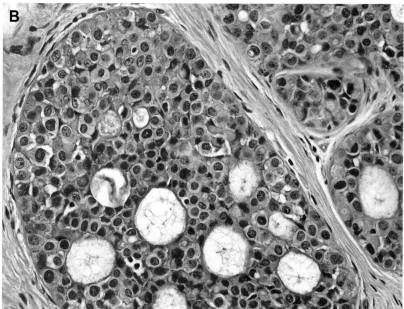

Fig. 9. Lobular carcinoma in situ, classical type (C-LCIS) involving collagenous spherulosis. (*A*) C-LCIS cells grow in between the spherules of collagenous spherulosis, simulating ductal carcinoma in situ, low grade (200×). (*B*) The globoid deposits of extracellular matrix characteristic of collagenous spherulosis show variable size. Intracytoplasmic mucin is present in C-LCIS cells (400×).

invasive lobular carcinoma, but subsequent studies led to the classification of C-LCIS as a risk factor. C-LCIS confers an increased long-term risk of subsequent invasive carcinoma[11–14] amounting to 8 to 10 fold that of the general population.[15,16] Studies showed that the risk is bilateral[14,17,18] and most invasive carcinomas that develop in patients with C-LCIS have ductal morphology. Hence, for a long time, C-LCIS has been considered a risk lesion.

This concept has been re-evaluated in recent years, based on multiple lines of evidence. C-LCIS is the only alteration present in association with invasive lobular carcinoma (ILC) in 31% to 98% of cases[19,20] and patients who have this lesion appear to develop ILC more frequently than

Fig. 9. (*C*) The myoepithelium around the spherules is positive for calponin. (*D*) The neoplastic cells in between the spherules are negative for E-cadherin, supporting lobular differentiation. Notice that residual ductal epithelium shows strong and linear membranous staining with E-cadherin. Discontinuous dot-like positivity for E-cadherin is present in the tendrils of myoepithelial cells (*C*, *D* 400×).

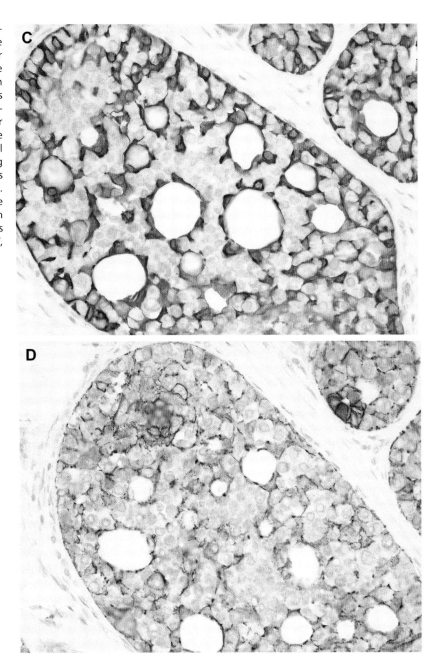

patients who do not.[19,20] When C-LCIS and ILC coexist, they are cytologically and immunophenotypically similar, if not identical. In addition, similar genetic alterations have been demonstrated in ILC and adjacent C-LCIS.[21,22] This evidence strongly suggests that C-LCIS is not only a marker of increased breast cancer risk, but likely represents a nonobligate precursor to ILC.[23] Progression of C-LCIS to ILC may occur at a lower rate than for ductal lesions and require more time to manifest. Until these issues are resolved, women with C-LCIS continue to be managed conservatively. No additional local therapy is recommended after C-LCIS is identified in a breast excision and presence of C-LCIS at or near margins is not commented upon. Tamoxifen decreases the risk of invasive carcinoma in women with C-LCIS[24] and it is routinely recommended for patients who have this lesion; alternatively, postmenopausal women with C-LCIS can receive aromatase inhibitors.

ATYPICAL LOBULAR HYPERPLASIA

ALH describes a neoplastic proliferation cytologically similar to C-LCIS but of relatively limited extent. Like C-LCIS, ALH has no specific clinical, radiologic, or macroscopic findings.

MICROSCOPIC FEATURES

The cells of ALH are monomorphic, small, round, or polygonal, with a thin rim of clear cytoplasm and high nuclear-to-cytoplasmic ratio. This morphology is indistinguishable from that of C-LCIS type A cells. In ALH, the neoplastic cells replace only a portion of the normal lobular epithelium, the terminal ductal lobular units are not completely distended, and few acinar lumina remain patent.

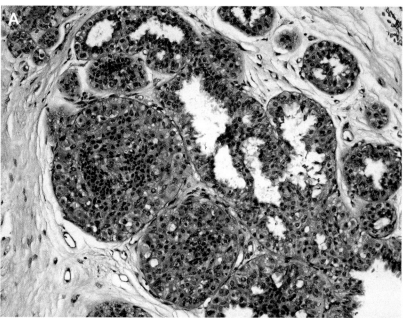

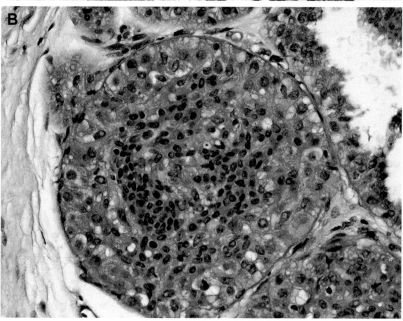

Fig. 10. Lobular carcinoma in situ, classical type (C-LCIS) involving usual ductal hyperplasia (UDH). (*A*) In this case, C-LCIS may be overlooked as UDH if the presence of a second population of cells at the periphery of the duct is not recognized (200×) (*B*) C-LCIS undermines UDH, lifting the cells toward the center of the duct. The lumen is completely occupied by a swirling population of cohesive ductal cells. Discohesive C-LCIS cells at the periphery of the duct are not polarized, and have slightly larger nuclei and pale cytoplasm.

DIAGNOSIS

As mentioned before, because the concept of complete distention of a lobule can be subjective, the distinction between ALH and C-LCIS remains loosely defined. Morphologic comparison with adjacent normal lobules uninvolved by lobular neoplasia is useful to determine the extent of relative distension. In 1978, Haagensen introduced the term lobular neoplasia (LN) to do away with the variability in diagnosis of C-LCIS and ALH[5]; and, more recently, Bratthauer and Tavassoli[25] proposed the designation of lobular intraepithelial neoplasia (LIN), but neither terminology is frequently used in common practice.

PROGNOSIS

The relative risk of subsequent breast cancer in women diagnosed with ALH is 4 to 5 fold higher than the risk of the general population,[15] whereas C-LCIS is 8 to 10 fold higher.[16] Therefore, although LN is a helpful collective term, specific classification into ALH and LCIS is preferable for risk stratification and patient management. Page and colleagues[26] reported that invasive carcinoma occurring in patients with prior diagnosis of ALH was about three times more likely to arise in the same breast as the index lesion than in the opposite breast. These data suggest a model of malignancy for ALH that is intermediate between a precursor and a generalized risk lesion.

MANAGEMENT OF C-LCIS OR ALH IDENTIFIED IN A CORE BIOPSY

No prospective data are available regarding the need to excise an area of the breast that has yielded C-LCIS or ALH on core needle biopsy. In such cases, excision is always required if mammographic and pathologic findings are discordant. Recently, Nagi and colleagues[27] reported the clinical follow-up of 98 subjects who had only C-LCIS or ALH on core biopsy. Only radiologic follow-up (range 1–8 years) was available for 48 subjects, all of whom were stable. Surgical excision was performed in 45 subjects and C-LCIS was the only lesion found in 42 of them. Only three subjects had a significant finding other than LN on surgical biopsy, including one with atypical ductal hyperplasia, one with DCIS and one with a focus of microinvasive lobular carcinoma. The investigators concluded that excision of lobular neoplasia is not required as long as careful radiographic–pathologic correlation is performed and strict diagnostic criteria are applied. Notably, the relative rate of lesion upgrade (microinvasive carcinoma

and DCIS) in the group of subjects who underwent excision amounted to 4%. In addition, these subjects did not show any radiologic abnormality, and this raises questions regarding the presence of more severe pathology in the subgroup of patients for which only radiologic follow-up was available. Cohen[28] reviewed 14 published studies reporting the findings in excisional biopsies from a total of 159 subjects diagnosed with C-LCIS or ALH in a core biopsy. The excision yielded DCIS or invasive carcinoma in about one in five of these subjects (30/159, 19%). Based on these findings, Cohen concluded that the diagnosis of LCIS and/or ALH in a core biopsy should be pursued with surgical excision. All available studies have been retrospective, and are limited by a selection bias because in the past not all patients with a diagnosis of C-LCIS on core biopsy underwent a subsequent excision.

IMMUNOPROFILE: LOBULAR NEOPLASIA: E-CADHERIN AND OTHER MARKERS

E-cadherin is a transmembrane glycoprotein involved in calcium-dependent, cell-to-cell adhesion. It is expressed mainly in epithelial cells and plays a critical role in epithelial differentiation and morphogenesis.[29,30] Studies on the molecular profile of breast carcinoma have consistently demonstrated that the E-cadherin gene (CDH1), located on chromosome 16q22.1, is deleted or mutated or epigenetically inactivated in lobular neoplasia, whereas it is maintained in ductal lesions.[31,32] This alteration results in loss of the extracellular domain of E-cadherin, detectable as lack of membranous immunoreactivity for this antigen. Loss of E-cadherin is an early event and is present in LCIS as well as in ALH.[33] The structural and/or functional loss of E-cadherin protein in lobular lesions likely contributes to the discohesive growth of the neoplastic cells.[34]

Strong linear membranous reactivity for E-cadherin decorates normal and neoplastic ductal cells, as well as normal lobular epithelium. The myoepithelium shows a characteristic discontinuous and granular pattern of membranous immunoreactivity. Several studies have demonstrated that E-cadherin immunoreactivity can reliably be used to distinguish ductal from lobular neoplasia (LCIS and ALH) (Fig. 11).[35,36]

In most cases, interpretation of E-cadherin staining is not problematic (positive or negative), but it can occasionally be challenging. Focal E-cadherin positivity in the tendrils of the myoepithelium admixed with LCIS may be attributed to the neoplastic cells, leading to misdiagnosis of DCIS. The dot-like, discontinuous, membranous staining

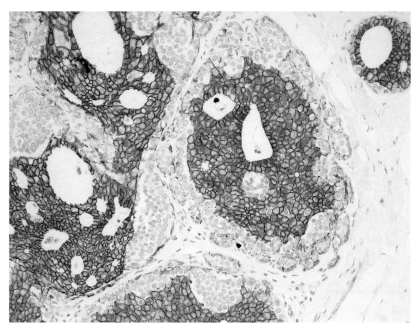

Fig. 11. Lobular carcinoma in situ, classical type (C-LCIS) and DCIS involving the same duct. Low-grade DCIS shows strong membranous staining for E-cadherin. C-LCIS cells are seen at the periphery of the duct, undermining DCIS, and lack membranous positivity for E-cadherin (200×).

of the attenuated myoepithelium needs to be distinguished from the strong and linear membranous positivity typical of the ductal cells. In these cases, it is important to assess E-cadherin immunoreactivity in small clusters of three or more neoplastic cells directly adjacent to each other, without interposed myoepithelium.

P120 catenin is the intracytoplasmic ligand of E-cadherin. Whenever E-cadherin is absent, the membrane bound p120 decreases whereas the cytoplasmic pool of free p120 increases. This change can be detected immunohistochemically.[37] Strong cytoplasmic positivity for p120 characterizes ALH as well as LCIS. In contrast, ductal proliferations show positive membranous immunoreactivity for p120.[38] At present p120 immunohistochemical stain is not widely applied.

High-molecular-weight cytokeratin (34βE12) can also aid in the differential diagnosis between ductal and lobular lesions. Neoplastic ductal lesions usually show no reactivity with 34βE12, whereas lobular neoplasia displays a characteristic cytoplasmic reaction, often in a distinct perinuclear pattern. Bratthauer and colleagues[39] found that the combination of E-cadherin and 34βE12 immunostain was very useful in distinguishing lobular and ductal lesions and clarified the nature of some cases with indeterminate morphology. In lobular and ductal neoplasia, a different staining pattern has also been reported for cytokeratin 8 (CK8). DCIS shows cytoplasmic positivity for CK8, with peripheral accentuation in foci of cell-to-cell contact, whereas a perinuclear staining

pattern is characteristic of lobular carcinoma.[40] The application of 34βE12 and CK8 immunoreactivity for the diagnosis of LCIS is also uncommon (**Table 2**).

C-LCIS is typically strongly ER positive and positive for PR in 60%–90% of cases. It rarely shows expression of HER2[41,42] or p53.[43,44] C-LCIS usually has no mitoses, and the MIB-1 proliferation index is low.

LOBULAR CARCINOMA IN SITU, SPECIAL VARIANTS

The widespread use of E-cadherin immunohistochemistry has greatly facilitated the categorization of a large number of morphologically ambiguous proliferations into ductal or lobular types. Its application has also revealed that a wide range of carcinomas in situ previously regarded as ductal lack membranous immunoreactivity for E-cadherin. These lesions have solid growth and consist of discohesive ovoid cells that fill up and expand the lumen of ducts and lobules, typically showing central necrosis and associated calcifications. The morphology of these lesions is vaguely reminiscent of that of C-LCIS, especially with regard to their discohesive growth, but nuclear atypia can range from moderate to severe, and mitoses are usually common. Classification of these in situ carcinomas remains problematic and there is no consensus on terminology. Herein, we refer to these lesions as "special types of LCIS" (S-LCIS) and subdivide them into two morphologic

Key Features
LOBULAR CARCINOMA IN SITU, SPECIAL TYPE

1. S-LCIS has morphologic features overlapping with those of DCIS and C-LCIS

2. S-LCIS consists of an E-cadherin negative solid and expansive proliferation of discohesive cells involving acini and ducts

3. The neoplastic cells are round-to-ovoid and can have abundant cytoplasm

4. Intracytoplasmic vacuoles and mucin are common, with signet ring cell formation

5. Central necrosis and mitoses are characteristic features of S-LCIS

6. S-LCIS can show marked nuclear pleomorphism

7. S-LCIS usually associates with invasive carcinoma and is rare in isolation

8. C-LCIS is often present at the periphery of S-LCIS

9. In the past, S-LCIS was classified as DCIS and treated as such

10. Outcome data for S-LCIS are very limited

11. Report any of these features of S-LCIS when present at or close to a margin:

   o Necrosis

   o Pleomorphic/signet ring cell morphology

   o Massive acinar/duct distention

   In these cases, re-excision should be considered.

subtypes: S-LCIS composed of type A and/or type B cells, and S-LCIS with pleomorphic nuclei. This nomenclature is used only for the purpose of description, and is not intended for nosologic classification.

GROSS FEATURES

Calcifications are frequently associated with S-LCIS and often lead to mammographic identification of these lesions. The involvement and expansion of acini and medium-sized ducts can sometimes be detected as an area of architectural distortion on a mammogram.

MICROSCOPIC FEATURES

The morphologic features of S-LCIS are usually most obvious in the central nidus of expanded and closely juxtaposed acini and ducts, where S-LCIS displays solid and expansile growth with central necrosis (**Fig. 12**). In S-LCIS, the cells fill up the entire lumen of a duct, completely obliterating it, in contrast to the persistence of a central, though compressed, lumen characteristic of C-LCIS with pagetoid involvement of ducts. The cytomorphology of S-LCIS also tends to be more severe in the central nidus of the lesion. The tumor cells are round-to-ovoid and discohesive. Loss of cohesion is readily appreciated around the central necrotic focus, but it is also evident throughout the rest of the lesion. Central necrosis is a qualifying feature of S-LCIS and frequently contains coarse calcifications. As a result, S-LCIS can be detected mammographically as pleomorphic calcifications with branching linear distribution, a pattern previously regarded as uniquely ductal. Mitoses are frequent, including abnormal ones. Apoptosis also occurs and histiocytes with abundant clear cytoplasm containing apoptotic debris are often scattered among the neoplastic cells. On low-power magnification the clear cytoplasm of large histiocytes may resemble the lumen of a cribriform space.

S-LCIS tends to form a discrete lesion, but at its periphery it often transitions into C-LCIS (**Fig. 13**). S-LCIS is very rarely observed as an isolated lesion, and it usually occurs in association with invasive carcinoma, most often of lobular type.[45,46]

Table 2			
Antigens useful to distinguish LCIS versus DCIS			
Antigens	**Normal distribution**	**LCIS**	**DCIS**
E-cadherin	Cell membrane	Absent[a]	Same as normal
p120 catenin	Cell membrane and cytoplasm	Loss on cell membrane, increased in cytoplasm	Same as normal
CK 34BE12	Cell membrane and cytoplasm	Perinuclear	Absent
CK 8	Cell membrane and cytoplasm	Perinuclear	Cytoplasm

CK, cytokeratin

[a] May show some faint cytoplasmic positivity in special variants of LCIS with pleomorphic nuclei.

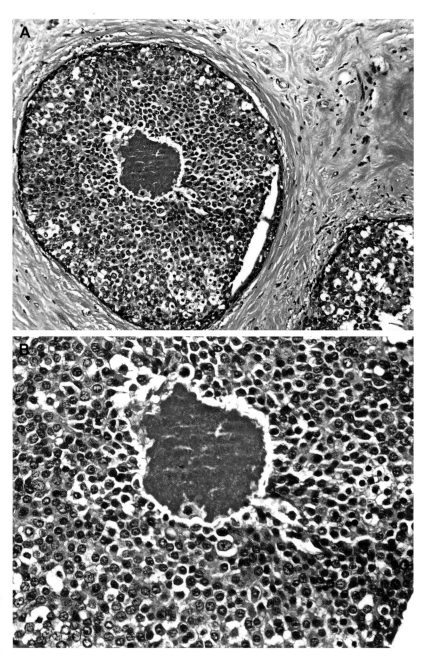

Fig. 12. Lobular carcinoma in situ, special type (S-LCIS) with central necrosis. (*A*) A duct is distended by a proliferation of small, loosely cohesive cells with central necrosis (100×). (*B*) The neoplastic cells display type A and type B morphology. Presence of necrosis and massive expansion of the duct differentiate this carcinoma from C-LCIS (400×).

Special Types of Lobular Carcinoma In Situ with Type A and Type B Cells

In these lesions the ducts are expanded and entirely filled by a population of small, round, inconspicuous cells with bland nuclei and scant cytoplasm (type A cells), whereas others show slightly larger cells with enlarged nuclei and visible nucleoli (type B cells). Some lesions show a mixture of type A and type B cells (**Fig. 14**).

Mitotic figures are usually apparent, as well as apoptotic bodies. Nuclear size can range from 1.5 to 2.5 times the size of a red blood cell. Some cells show signet ring cell morphology.

Special Types of Lobular Carcinoma In Situ with Pleomorphic Nuclei

The neoplastic cells are large and have ample-to-abundant cytoplasm and enlarged nuclei, often

Fig. 13. Lobular carcinoma in situ, special type (S-LCIS) with central necrosis expands ducts and acini. (*A*) The florid expansion of closely juxtaposed acini and ducts involved by S-LCIS contrasts with the relatively lower degree of enlargement of adjacent lobules involved by C-LCIS. (*B*) In this case, the S-LCIS cells have similar nuclei but slightly more abundant cytoplasm than the cells of the adjacent C-LCIS.

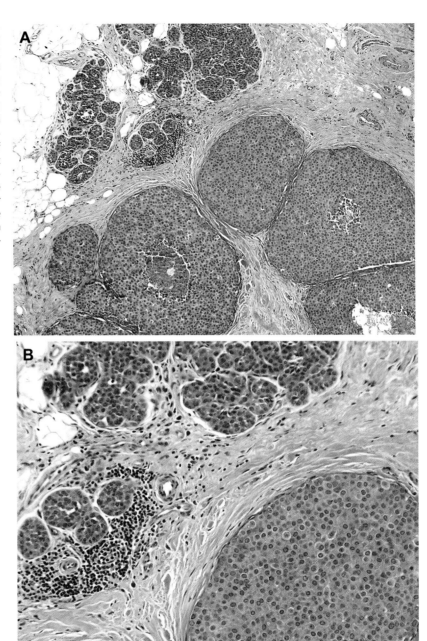

pleomorphic, with prominent nucleoli (**Fig 15**). Sometimes the tumor cells resting on the basement membrane are much larger than those located in the center of the duct/acinus, and show higher-grade morphology. The nucleus is often shifted to one pole of the cell, resulting in a plasmacytoid appearance (**Fig 16**). Accumulation of intracytoplasmic mucin can occur, imparting a blue-gray hue to the cell. Mucin can be so abundant to indent and displace the nucleus, with resulting signet ring cell morphology. In some cases, the cytoplasm is very pale, foamy, and fragile, and the cells resemble foamy histiocytes, but the nuclear atypia is severe (**Fig 17**). Large cells with densely eosinophilic cytoplasm can also occur, and show apocrine features. At the extreme end of the spectrum, S-LCIS with pleomorphic nuclei is composed of cells with large nuclei (about 3 to 4 times the size of a red blood cell) that have an irregular nuclear membrane and coarse nuclear chromatin. Nucleoli are easily identified, can be multiple, and have abnormal

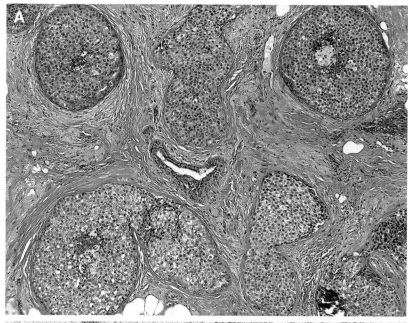

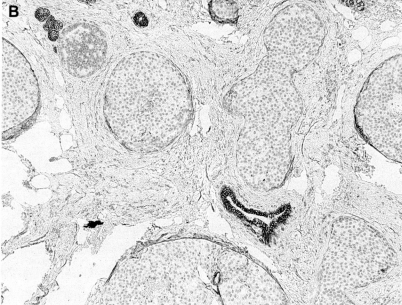

Fig. 14. Lobular carcinoma in situ, special type, (S-LCIS) with type A and type B cells is negative for E-cadherin. (*A*) The ducts are expanded by a solid proliferation of small cells and show central necrosis. (*B*) The tumor cells lack membranous immunoreactivity for E-cadherin, confirming a lobular phenotype. A duct uninvolved by S-LCIS shows strong immunoreactivity for the same antigen.

shape. Binucleate cells are also common, especially in pleomorphic S-LCIS with apocrine features. S-LCIS with pleomorphic nuclei can sometimes show some cytoplasmic positivity for E-cadherin.

DIFFERENTIAL DIAGNOSIS

In all its possible cytomorphologic variants, S-LCIS with central necrosis very closely resembles DCIS. Lack of cell cohesion, round-to-ovoid morphology, presence of intracytoplasmic lumina, and/or abundant intracytoplasmic mucin are morphologic features that favor lobular over ductal differentiation. Lack of membranous immunoreactivity for E-cadherin provides additional confirmatory evidence of lobular differentiation. Nonetheless, until very recently, S-LCIS was classified as DCIS and managed as such. This important information must always be

Fig. 15. Lobular carcinoma in situ, special type (S-LCIS) with pleomorphic nuclei. (*A*) Few ducts and acini are expanded by a proliferation of large and discohesive cells. A coarse calcification is present. (*B*) The neoplastic cells show enlarged and pleomorphic nuclei and intracytoplasmic vacuoles.

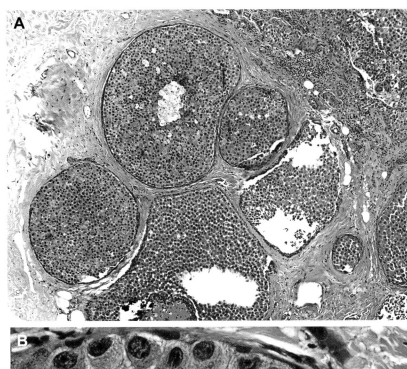

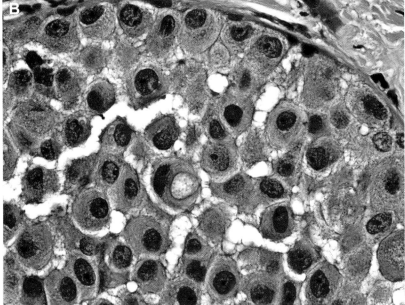

communicated and discussed with the treating clinicians, especially if no invasive carcinoma is associated with S-LCIS.

PROGNOSIS

Studies on S-LCIS are very few and retrospective, with limited follow-up data. This is not surprising given that S-LCIS is rare as an isolated lesion. Its frequent association with invasive carcinoma suggests that S-LCIS is more aggressive than C-LCIS, as also indicated by the presence of necrosis and frequent mitoses.

Fadare and colleagues[45] reviewed 18 subjects who had LCIS with comedo-type necrosis. In these cases the cells showed either type A and/ or type B morphology. All cases lacked membranous reactivity for E-cadherin. LCIS with comedo-type necrosis consisted of a solid proliferation distending the acini to variable degree; comedo-

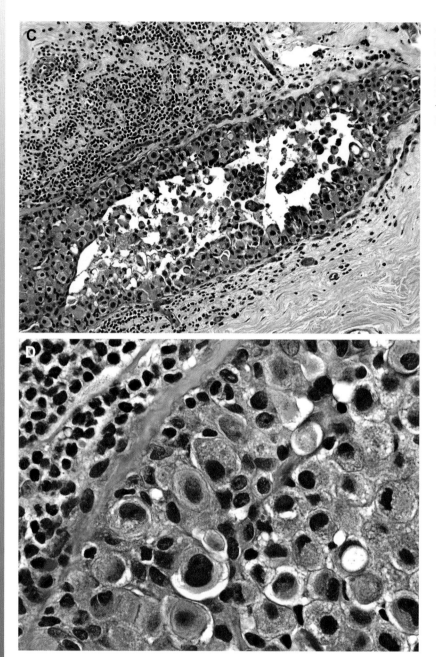

Fig. 15. (*C*) The tumor displays discohesive growth. (*D*) Binucleate cells are often seen in S-LCIS with pleomorphic nuclei. Nuclei are three times the size of adjacent lymphocytes.

type necrosis was focal to extensive. The cells were loosely cohesive and regularly spaced, had small-to-intermediate size and round or polygonal shape, and showed high nuclear-to-cytoplasmic ratio. All these lesions were devoid of significant nuclear pleomorphism. Invasive carcinoma was present in 12 (67%) of 18 cases, and had lobular morphology in eleven (seven classical, one pleomorphic, one hybrid ductal lobular, one tubular with minor lobular component, and one with lobular and ductal carcinoma as separate foci),

and pure ductal in one. Calcifications were present in 10 (55%) of 18 cases, and typically occurred within the necrotic foci. Nearly all tumors (17/18 cases) were positive for high-molecular-weight keratin and ER, and HER2/neu negative (15/18 cases). The investigators noted that LCIS with comedo-type necrosis occurred at an older age (62.5 years) than classic LCIS (52 years) and was commonly associated with invasive carcinoma, which was more frequently lobular than ductal.

Fig. 16. Lobular carcinoma in situ, special type with pleomorphic nuclei. The neoplastic cells have abundant eosinophilic cytoplasm and large nuclei with conspicuous nucleoli. A mitotic figure is present.

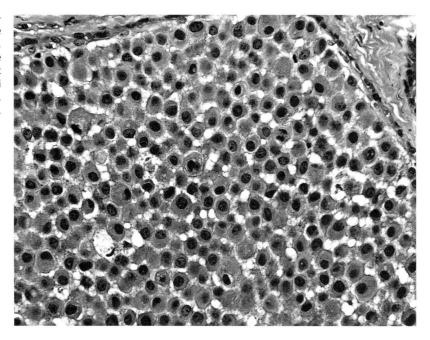

Sneige and colleagues[46] examined cases of LCIS with pleomorphic features, designated as pleomorphic–lobular/ductal–lobular carcinoma in situ (PL/DLCIS). Their study cases consisted of 10 pure PL/DLCIS and 14 PL/DLCIS associated with invasive pleomorphic lobular carcinoma. Histologically, PL/DLCIS cells were discohesive, had intermediate-to-large size, moderate-to-marked nuclear pleomorphism, small-to-prominent nucleoli, and moderate-to-abundant eosinophilic or vacuolated cytoplasm. Central necrosis was present in 40% of pure PL/DLCIS and in 12% PL/DLCIS associated with invasion. C-LCIS coexisted with PL/DCIS in 10 of 24 cases [4 PL/DLCIS and 6 PL/DLCIS cases with invasion]. E-cadherin was negative in all cases. All PL/DLCIS were positive for ER (100%), six for p53 (25%), and 14 for GCDFP-15 (74%). HER-2/neu gene amplification was observed in only one (4%) of 23 cases. Seven of the 10 subjects with pure PL/DLCIS underwent lumpectomy or simple mastectomy, and six had no evidence of

Fig. 17. Lobular carcinoma in situ, special type with pleomorphic nuclei and histiocytoid type cells. In the center of the duct, true histiocytes are seen with abundant clear cytoplasm containing apoptotic debris. On low-power magnification the clear cytoplasm of large histiocytes may resemble the lumen of a cribriform space, but closer examination reveals the true nature of these spaces.

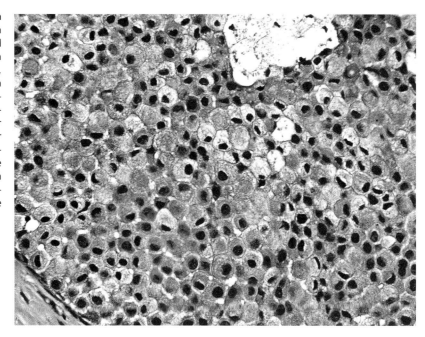

Differential Diagnosis
LOBULAR CARCINOMA IN SITU,
SPECIAL TYPES

Special types of lobular carcinoma in situ

- Ductal Carcinoma in situ, intermediate to high nuclear grade

  o Cell polarity and focal microacini support ductal differentiation

  o DCIS cells show a polygonal outline and distinct cytoplasmic borders.

  o In contrast to DCIS, LCIS shows discohesive cells, intracytoplasmic "targetoid inclusions," and more frequently associated pagetoid involvement of ducts.

  o Use E-cadherin to resolve problematic cases.

disease in follow-up periods ranging from 4 to 32 months; the seventh patient developed suspicious calcifications 12 months after the index biopsy and was diagnosed with recurrent PL/DLCIS.

Chivukula and colleagues[47] recently studied 12 cases of S-LCIS with pleomorphic features (referred to as P-LCIS) diagnosed on core needle biopsy and the findings in the subsequent surgical excision. Lobular differentiation was confirmed by negative E-cadherin and cytoplasmic-dominant staining with p120 catenin in all cases. P-LCIS was positive for ER in 11 (92%) cases and for HER2/neu in three (25%). Moderate to high proliferative activity was observed with MIB (Ki-67) staining in 92% (11/12) cases. Residual P-LCIS was found in the follow-up excision in 10 (83%) subjects and invasive lobular carcinoma in three (25%).

There is uniform consensus that if S-LCIS is identified in a core biopsy, the lesion needs to be entirely excised. Similarly, re-excision is recommended when S-LCIS with acinar distention, and/or necrosis, and/or pleomorphic signet ring cell morphology is found close by or at a surgical margin.[7] Some pathologists still prefer to categorize S-LCIS as in situ carcinoma with ductal and lobular features rather than as variants of LCIS (**Table 3**). At present, there is no consensus on whether patients who have S-LCIS treated with breast conservation should also undergo radiotherapy. Long-term follow-up studies are needed to better define the natural history of S-LCIS and its optimal management.

CARCINOMA IN SITU OF INDETERMINATE FEATURES

Currently most in situ carcinomas of the breast are easily categorized as either DCIS or LCIS; however, lesions with intermediate morphology can occur albeit rarely. In some in situ carcinomas with solid morphology, the cytologic or architectural features deviate from the usual patterns, making it difficult to determine if the proliferation is ductal or lobular. Occasionally, even the pattern of immunostaining shows inconclusive results. A carcinoma in situ with indeterminate features (CIS-IF) usually consists of a solid proliferation of cells showing no polarity and variable degree of E-cadherin positivity (**Fig. 18**).

Jacobs and colleagues[48] looked at the E-cadherin expression in a series of cases of mammary CIS-IF in an attempt to better categorize the lesions as ductal or lobular. They divided the lesions into three groups. Group 1 had all of the cytologic and architectural features typical of LCIS but exhibited areas of comedo-type central necrosis. Group 2 consisted of in situ carcinoma that had some features of DCIS and some of LCIS. Group 3 exhibited growth patterns characteristic of LCIS but cytologic features similar to high grade DCIS (similar to cases reported as pleomorphic lobular carcinoma in situ [PLCIS]). All cases in groups 1 and 3 were E-cadherin–negative akin to LCIS. According to the nomenclature we have used in this discussion, group 1 would fall in the category of S-LCIS with type A or type B cells, group 3 in the category of S-LCIS with pleomorphic cells. Group 2 lesions were

Table 3 Terminology commonly used for reporting of S-LCIS	
Special LCIS with type A and type B cells	Lobular neoplasia with comedo necrosis[45] Carcinoma with mixed ductal and lobular features Carcinoma with indeterminate features[48]
Special LCIS with pleomorphic nuclei	Pleomorphic LCIS[51] Carcinoma with mixed ductal and lobular features

Fig. 18. Ductal carcinoma in situ with a focus showing indeterminate features. (*A*) Solid proliferation of neoplastic cells expands few ducts and lobules. (*B*) This proliferation is E-cadherin positive, and qualifies as ductal carcinoma in situ; however, a duct shows a gradation in staining intensity (*A*, *B* 100×)

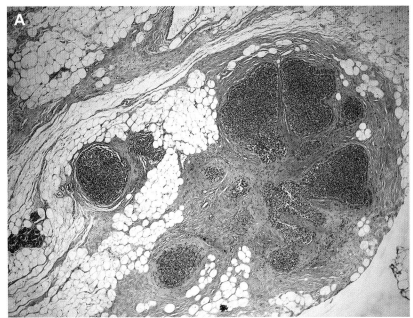

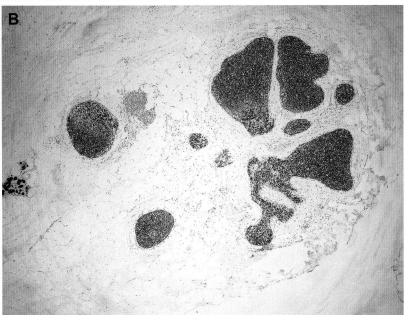

heterogeneous with respect to E-cadherin staining, with 35% E-cadherin–negative and 30% E-cadherin–positive, suggesting ductal phenotype. The final 35% had both E-cadherin–positive and E-cadherin–negative tumor cells. suggesting a mixed ductal/lobular phenotype. The investigators concluded that E-cadherin immunohistochemistry is a valuable adjunct in the categorization of carcinoma in situ lesions, with E-cadherin–negative lesions best considered lobular, and E-cadherin–positive lesions best considered ductal. Proliferations showing a mixed staining pattern should be considered as mixed ductal/lobular lesions.

Da Silva and colleagues[49] reported cases of ILC with aberrant positive E-cadherin immunoreactivity. Among them were carcinomas with heterogeneous E-cadherin expression and some with weak E-cadherin positivity, suggestive of ductal phenotype. These cases had an in-frame

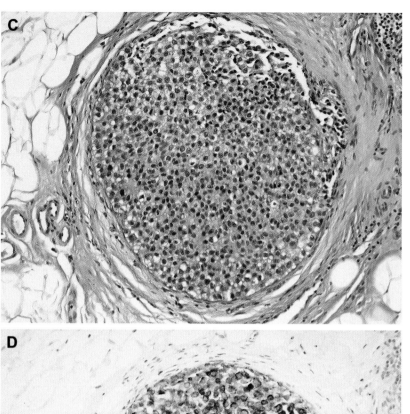

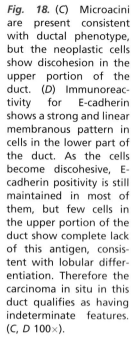

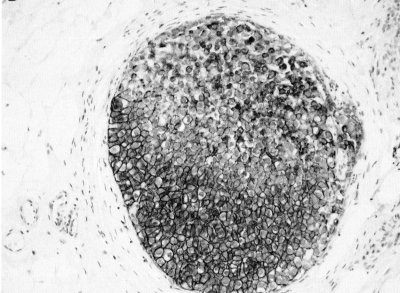

Fig. 18. (*C*) Microacini are present consistent with ductal phenotype, but the neoplastic cells show discohesion in the upper portion of the duct. (*D*) Immunoreactivity for E-cadherin shows a strong and linear membranous pattern in cells in the lower part of the duct. As the cells become discohesive, E-cadherin positivity is still maintained in most of them, but few cells in the upper portion of the duct show complete lack of this antigen, consistent with lobular differentiation. Therefore the carcinoma in situ in this duct qualifies as having indeterminate features. (*C, D* 100×).

deletion of the E-cadherin gene and loss of the wild-type allele. In these cases, the dysfunctional E-cadherin protein was present but did not bind the catenin complex. They concluded that some carcinomas with lobular morphology express a nonfunctional form of E-cadherin and will still retain some positivity for this antigen. In their opinion, positive staining for E-cadherin should not preclude a diagnosis of lobular carcinoma if the tumor shows typical morphology.

Recent studies by Ellis[19,50] and his group have shown a close relationship between C-LCIS, ALH, columnar cell changes, atypical ductal hyperplasia, low-grade DCIS and low-grade invasive carcinomas (tubular carcinoma, invasive lobular carcinoma, and invasive ductal carcinoma with low nuclear grade). Based on morphologic, immunophenotypic, and molecular evidence, Ellis and colleagues have proposed a unified view of these lesions as related forms of low-grade mammary neoplasia. This novel hypothesis provides a possible explanation for CIS-IF as a low-grade carcinoma in situ bridging low-grade DCIS and C-LCIS. To date, no study has suggested a relationship between S-LCIS and DCIS.

Clinical outcome data are lacking for lesions that fall under CIS-IF and, due to their rarity, it may be difficult to accrue enough cases for a study. Some pathologists may use the diagnosis of DCIS only, or carcinoma with mixed ductal and lobular features, or diagnose DCIS *and* LCIS. All of these diagnoses are acceptable. For the practical purpose of patient management, it is important to convey to the clinician the information that CIS-IF displays ductal features to ensure that the patient is managed accordingly.

SUMMARY

LCIS is a heterogeneous disease both clinically and morphologically. For many years, LCIS has been regarded as a marker lesion of increased risk for invasive carcinoma. Recent evidence, however, suggests that LCIS represents a nonobligate precursor to invasive carcinoma. The progression of LCIS to invasion appears to be less frequent and slower than for DCIS. With the application of E-cadherin, pathologists have learned to recognize unusual variants of LCIS that were previously categorized as ductal carcinoma. The appropriate treatment of S-LCIS is

currently debated as information on the clinical outcome remains very limited at present.

REFERENCES

1. Foote F, Stewart F. Lobular carcinoma in situ. A rare form of mammary cancer. Am J Clin Pathol 1941;17: 491–5.
2. Li CI, Anderson BO, Daling JR, et al. Changing incidence of lobular carcinoma in situ of the breast. Breast Cancer Res Treat 2002;75(3):259–68.
3. Pope TL Jr, Fechner RE, Wilhelm MC, et al. Lobular carcinoma in situ of the breast: mammographic features. Radiology 1988;168(1):63–6.
4. Brogi E, Oyama T, Koerner FC. Atypical cystic lobules in patients with lobular neoplasia. Int J Surg Pathol 2001;9(3):201–6.
5. Haagensen CD, Lane N, Lattes R, et al. Lobular neoplasia (so-called lobular carcinoma in situ) of the breast. Cancer 1978;42(2):737–69.
6. Azzopardi JG. Problems in breast pathology. Philadelphia: Saunders; 1979.
7. Tavassoli FA, Devilee P, editors. World Health Organization classification of tumors. Pathology and genetics of the female genital organs. Lobular neoplasia, Lyon (France): IARC Press; 2003. p. 60–2.
8. Ozzello L. Ultrastructure of intra-epithelial carcinomas of the breast. Cancer 1971;28(6):1508–15.
9. Page DL, Anderson TJ. Diagnostic Histopathology of the Breast. New York: Churchill Livingstone; 1987.
10. Rosen PP. Lobular carcinoma in situ and intraductal carcinoma of the breast. In: McDivitt RW, Oberman HA, Ozzello L, Kaufman N, editors. The breast. Baltimore (MD): Williams and Wilkins; 1984. p. 59–105.
11. Page DL, Kidd TE Jr, Dupont WD, et al. Lobular neoplasia of the breast: higher risk for subsequent invasive cancer predicted by more extensive disease. Hum Pathol 1991;22(12):1232–9.
12. Rosen PP, Kosloff C, Lieberman PH, et al. Lobular carcinoma in situ of the breast. Detailed analysis of 99 patients with average follow-up of 24 years. Am J Surg Pathol 1978;2(3):225–51.
13. Nielsen M, Jensen J, Andersen J. Precancerous and cancerous breast lesions during lifetime and at autopsy. A study of 83 women. Cancer 1984;54(4):612–5.
14. Rosen PP, Braun DW Jr, Lyngholm B, et al. Lobular carcinoma in situ of the breast: preliminary results of treatment by ipsilateral mastectomy and contralateral breast biopsy. Cancer 1981;47(4):813–9.
15. Page DL, Dupont WD. Anatomic markers of human premalignancy and risk of breast cancer. Cancer 1990;66(6 Suppl):1326–35.
16. Page DL, Dupont WD, Rogers LW, et al. Atypical hyperplastic lesions of the female breast. A long term follow-up study. Cancer 1985;55(11):2698–708.

Pitfalls
LOBULAR CARCINOMA IN SITU, CLASSICAL TYPE

! Ductal carcinoma in situ, low grade, extending into lobules may closely resemble C-LCIS.

- Focal acinar arrangement favors DCIS
- Columnar cell morphology favors DCIS. This feature is more evident in the cells resting on the basement membrane
- Polygonal cells with sharply defined cell membrane are typical of DCIS, but not specific

! C- LCIS involving collagenous spherulosis can simulate cribriform DCIS

Note: The diagnostic differential between C-LCIS and low-grade DCIS should always be pursued, as management of these two lesions differs greatly

17. Rosen PP, Senie R, Schottenfeld D, et al. Noninvasive breast carcinoma: frequency of unsuspected invasion and implications for treatment. Ann Surg 1979;189(3):377–82.

18. Urban JA. Bilaterality of cancer of the breast. Biopsy of the opposite breast. Cancer 1967;20(11):1867–70.

19. Abdel-Fatah TM, Powe DG, Hodi Z, et al. High frequency of coexistence of columnar cell lesions, lobular neoplasia, and low grade ductal carcinoma in situ with invasive tubular carcinoma and invasive lobular carcinoma. Am J Surg Pathol 2007;31(3):417–26.

20. Wheeler JE, Enterline HT, Roseman JM, et al. Lobular carcinoma in situ of the breast. Long-term followup. Cancer 1974;34(3):554–63.

21. Berx G, Cleton-Jansen AM, Strumane K, et al. E-cadherin is inactivated in a majority of invasive human lobular breast cancers by truncation mutations throughout its extracellular domain. Oncogene 1996;13(9):1919–25.

22. Vos CB, Cleton-Jansen AM, Berx G, et al. E-cadherin inactivation in lobular carcinoma in situ of the breast: an early event in tumorigenesis. Br J Cancer 1997;76(9):1131–3.

23. Lishman SC, Lakhani SR. Atypical lobular hyperplasia and lobular carcinoma in situ: surgical and molecular pathology. Histopathology 1999;35(3):195–200.

24. Fisher B, Costantino JP, Wickerham DL, et al. Tamoxifen for prevention of breast cancer: report of the National Surgical Adjuvant Breast and Bowel Project P-1 Study. J Natl Cancer Inst 1998;90(18):1371–88.

25. Bratthauer GL, Tavassoli FA. Lobular intraepithelial neoplasia: previously unexplored aspects assessed in 775 cases and their clinical implications. Virchows Arch 2002;440(2):134–8.

26. Page DL, Schuyler PA, Dupont WD, et al. Atypical lobular hyperplasia as a unilateral predictor of breast cancer risk: a retrospective cohort study. Lancet 2003;361:125–9.

27. Nagi CS, O'Donnell JE, Tismenetsky M, et al. Lobular neoplasia on core needle biopsy does not require excision. Cancer 2008;112(10):2152–8.

28. Cohen MA. Cancer upgrades at excisional biopsy after diagnosis of atypical lobular hyperplasia or lobular carcinoma in situ at core-needle biopsy: some reasons why. Radiology 2004;231(3):617–21.

29. Gumbiner BM. Regulation of cadherin adhesive activity. J Cell Biol 2000;148(3):399–404.

30. Deman JJ, Van Larebeke NA, Bruyneel EA, et al. Removal of sialic acid from the surface of human MCF-7 mammary cancer cells abolishes E-cadherin-dependent cell-cell adhesion in an aggregation assay. In Vitro Cell Dev Biol Anim 1995;31(8):633–9.

31. Etzell JE, Devries S, Florendo C, et al. Loss of chromosome 16q in lobular carcinoma in situ. Human Pathology 2001;32(3):292–6.

32. Berx G, Cleton-Jansen AM, Strumane K, et al. E-cadherin is inactivated in a majority of invasive human lobular breast cancers by truncation mutations through its extracellular domain. Oncogene 1996;13:1919–25.

33. Mastracci TL, Tjan S, Bane AL, et al. E-cadherin alterations in atypical lobular hyperplasia and lobular carcinoma in situ of the breast. Mod Pathol 2005;18(6):741–51.

34. Kowalski PJ, Rubin MA, Kleer CG. E-cadherin expression in primary carcinomas of the breast and its distant metastases. Breast Cancer Res 2003;5(6):R217–22.

35. Acs G, Lawton TJ, Rebbeck TR, et al. Differential expression of E-cadherin in lobular and ductal neoplasms of the breast and its biologic and diagnostic implications. Am J Clin Pathol 2001;115(1):85–98.

36. Moll R, Mitze M, Frixen UH, et al. Differential loss of E-cadherin expression in infiltrating ductal and lobular breast carcinomas. Am J Pathol 1993;143(6):1731–42.

37. Sarrio D, Perez-Mies B, Hardisson D, et al. Cytoplasmic localization of p120ctn and E-cadherin loss characterize lobular breast carcinoma from preinvasive to metastatic lesions. Oncogene 2004;23(19):3272–83.

38. Dabbs DJ, Bhargava R, Chivukula M. Lobular versus ductal breast neoplasms: the diagnostic utility of p120 catenin. Am J Surg Pathol 2007;31(3):427–37.

39. Bratthauer GL, Moinfar F, Stamatakos MD, et al. Combined E-cadherin and high molecular weight cytokeratin immunoprofile differentiates lobular, ductal, and hybrid mammary intraepithelial neoplasias. Hum Pathol 2002;33(6):620–7.

40. Lehr HA, Folpe A, Yaziji H, et al. Cytokeratin 8 immunostaining pattern and E-cadherin expression distinguish lobular from ductal breast carcinoma. Am J Clin Pathol 2000;114(2):190–6.

41. Ramachandra S, Machin L, Ashley S, et al. Immunohistochemical distribution of c-erbB-2 in in situ breast carcinoma–a detailed morphological analysis. J Pathol 1990;161(1):7–14.

42. Somerville JE, Clarke LA, Biggart JD. c-erbB-2 overexpression and histological type of in situ and invasive breast carcinoma. J Clin Pathol 1992;45(1):16–20.

43. Mohsin SK, O'Connell P, Allred DC, et al. Biomarker profile and genetic abnormalities in lobular carcinoma in situ. Breast Cancer Res Treat 2005;90(3):249–56.

44. Rudas M, Neumayer R, Gnant MF, et al. p53 protein expression, cell proliferation and steroid hormone receptors in ductal and lobular in situ carcinomas of the breast. Eur J Cancer 1997;33(1):39–44.

45. Fadare O, Dadmanesh F, Alvarado-Cabrero I, et al. Lobular intraepithelial neoplasia [lobular carcinoma

in situ] with comedo-type necrosis: a clinicopathologic study of 18 cases. Am J Surg Pathol 2006; 30(11):1445–53.

46. Sneige N, Wang J, Baker BA, et al. Clinical, histopathologic, and biologic features of pleomorphic lobular (ductal-lobular) carcinoma in situ of the breast: a report of 24 cases. Mod Pathol 2002; 15(10):1044–50.

47. Chivukula M, Haynik DM, Brufsky A, et al. Pleomorphic lobular carcinoma in situ (PLCIS) on breast core needle biopsies: clinical significance and immunoprofile. Am J Surg Pathol 2008; 32(11):1721–6.

48. Jacobs TW, Pliss N, Kouria G, et al. Carcinomas in situ of the breast with indeterminate features: role of E-cadherin staining in categorization. Am J Surg Pathol 2001;25(2):229–36.

49. Da Silva L, Parry S, Reid L, et al. Aberrant expression of E-cadherin in lobular carcinomas of the breast. Am J Surg Pathol 2008;32(5):773–83.

50. Abdel-Fatah TM, Powe DG, Hodi Z, et al. Morphologic and molecular evolutionary pathways of low nuclear grade invasive breast cancers and their putative precursor lesions: further evidence to support the concept of low nuclear grade breast neoplasia family. Am J Surg Pathol 2008;32(4): 513–23.

51. Frost A, Tsangaris T, Silverberg S. Pleomorphic lobular carcinoma in situ. Pathol Case Rev 1996; 1(1):27–31.

UPDATE ON FIBROEPITHELIAL LESIONS OF THE BREAST

Timothy W. Jacobs, MD

KEYWORDS

• Phyllodes tumor • Fibroepithelial • Fibroadenoma • Breast core biopsy • Cellular fibroadenoma

ABSTRACT

This article focuses on current issues relating to fibroepithelial lesions, predominantly those with cellular stroma, and covers key pathologic features, differential diagnosis, and pitfalls. Phyllodes tumors are emphasized, including the histologic categorization and prognostic features of these lesions. The management of fibroepithelial lesions on needle core biopsy is reviewed.

Cellular fibroepithelial lesions encompass a spectrum of entities, ranging from cellular fibroadenoma to phyllodes tumor. These lesions are diagnostically challenging for practicing pathologists and present management issues for breast imagers and clinicians alike. In contrast, morphologically classic fibroadenomas present few diagnostic or management dilemmas and are only briefly covered here (for an excellent recent review, see Lerwill[1]). This update concentrates primarily on the differential diagnosis of cellular fibroepithelial lesions, with particular emphasis on phyllodes tumors and their distinction from cellular fibroadenoma. In addition, the pathologic categorization of phyllodes tumors, prognostic features, and the use of marker studies are discussed. Lastly, management issues pertaining to cellular fibroepithelial lesions on core biopsy are covered.

FIBROADENOMA

OVERVIEW AND TERMINOLOGY

Fibroadenomas are characterized by stromal and epithelial components. The stromal component consists of connective tissue similar in appearance and cellularity to normal perilobular stroma. In older lesions, the stroma may become hyalinized and may be calcified. The stroma may contain heterologous benign components such as mature adipose tissue or smooth muscle; however, their presence has no clinical significance. The epithelial component consists of well-defined glandlike and ductlike spaces lined by bland epithelial cells. Varying degrees of epithelial hyperplasia may be seen. Although of no clinical significance, the term "intracanalicular" has been used for fibroadenomas in which the stromal component compresses the glands into slitlike spaces; "pericanalicular" is used for fbibroadenomas in which the glandular structures have a rounded configuration; these patterns often coexist in the same lesion (**Fig. 1**). The term "complex fibroadenoma" has been used for those lesions that contain cysts larger than 3 mm in diameter, sclerosing adenosis, epithelial calcifications, or papillary apocrine change. In a follow-up

Key Features
USEFUL FOR CATEGORIZATION OF PHYLLODES TUMOR

- Stromal cellularity (moderate or marked)
- Stromal cell pleomorphism (minimal, moderate, or marked)
- Stromal mitotic count (per 10 high power fields: low <5, moderate 5–10, high >10)
- Lesional border (relatively circumscribed or frankly invasive)
- Stromal overgrowth (only stroma in a ×40 total field = ×4 objective and ×10 ocular)
- Heterologous sarcomatous elements (ie, other than fibrosarcoma)

Department of Pathology, Virginia Mason Medical Center, 1100 Ninth Avenue, Seattle, WA 98101, USA
E-mail address: Timothy.Jacobs@vmmc.org

Surgical Pathology 2 (2009) 301–317
doi:10.1016/j.path.2009.02.006

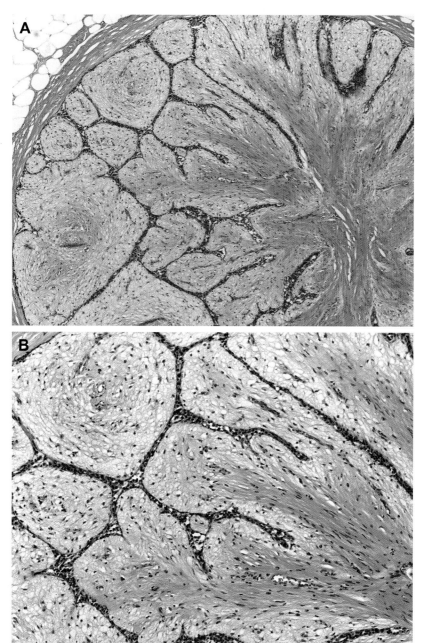

Fig. 1. Fibroadenoma. This lesion demonstrates an intracanalicular growth pattern in which the stromal component compresses glands in to slitlike spaces. The stroma is similar in appearance and cellularity to normal perilobular stroma. Note the well-circumscribed border. (A) ×40. (B) ×100.

study of 1835 patients, complex fibroadenomas were reported to be associated with a greater subsequent breast cancer risk than noncomplex fibroadenomas.[2] In a recent study, 63 of 401 (15.7%) consecutive fibroadenomas had complex features.[3] Although complex fibroadenomas tended to be smaller and occur in older patients, these investigators found a low incidence of associated malignancy. The designation of fibroadenoma as "complex" is not generally advocated in routine clinical practice. The term "giant fibroadenoma" has been used for otherwise histologically typical fibroadenomas that grow to a large size. This term has no specific clinical significance, and it is important to note that a large lesion with the microscopic features of conventional fibroadenoma should not be diagnosed as "benign phyllodes tumor" just because of its size, in the absence of features diagnostic of the latter (in particular, cellular stroma). Although most fibroadenomas in adolescents and younger women are of the usual type seen in older patients, some present a different clinical and pathologic picture and have been termed "juvenile fibroadenomas."[4–7] This entity has been used differently by some investigators, for example, to describe lesions that grow rapidly, with more glandular structures and cellular stroma,[4–6] and by other investigators for lesions that show severe epithelial hyperplasia that may border on carcinoma in situ.[7] It is important that these entities not be confused with phyllodes tumor, diagnostically and in communication with clinical colleagues.

PHYLLODES TUMORS

OVERVIEW

It is important to note that phyllodes tumors are uncommon lesions, accounting for approximately 0.3% to 1% of breast tumors in several series from tertiary referral centers (where the demographics are inherently skewed).[8–13] The true incidence in community practice is difficult to accurately gauge but is almost certainly far lower. In one community-based study, the Nottingham group identified a low frequency, with 32 phyllodes tumors compared with 6000 breast cancers over 15 years.[14] Phyllodes tumors account for approximately 2.5% of all fibroepithelial lesions.[13] Although the average age of presentation is often reported to be 40 to 50 years (approximately 15–20 years older than for fibroadenoma), phyllodes tumors have been reported to occur over a wider age range of 10 to 80 years.[11,13,15] Therefore, occurrence in a younger patient does not exclude the diagnosis.

GROSS FEATURES

On gross examination, phyllodes tumors are often well-circumscribed with a white, tan firm, bulging cut surface, and are therefore usually indistinguishable from fibroadenomas clinically and radiologically.[16–21] Clefts and cystlike spaces may sometimes be seen in larger lesions. Areas of hemorrhage and necrosis may be seen. Although an invasive tumor border is a useful diagnostic feature, this is not commonly recognized on gross inspection. The average size traditionally reported is 4 to 5 cm; however, due to the impact of mammographic screening, smaller tumors (1.3 to 3 cm) have been detected.[15,16,22] Size is therefore not a useful discriminatory feature between phyllodes tumor and fibroadenoma.

MICROSCOPIC FEATURES

The classic description of phyllodes tumor is that of a fibroepithelial lesion with cellular stroma (FELCS) and an enhanced intracanalicular growth pattern forming clefts or cystlike spaces. Leaflike projections of cellular stroma surfaced by epithelium protrude into these spaces (**Fig. 2**). Phyllodes tumors, however, encompass a spectrum of lesions. At one end are benign phyllodes tumors characterized by moderate stromal cellularity and minimal nuclear pleomorphism for which the distinction from fibroadenoma may be challenging. At the other end are frankly malignant-appearing spindle cell lesions with markedly cellular stroma, stromal cell pleomorphism, and easily identified mitotic figures (**Fig. 3**) for which the differential diagnosis is with sarcomatoid metaplastic carcinoma or sarcoma.

Differential Diagnosis of Phyllodes Tumor and Fibroadenoma

The main distinguishing feature between benign phyllodes tumor and fibroadenoma is the degree of stromal cellularity. In phyllodes tumors, the stroma is more cellular and the stromal cells appear more closely packed. In conjunction, the cleft and leaflike pattern of phyllodes tumor is characteristically present. Fibroadenomas are well-circumscribed grossly and microscopically (**Fig. 4**), whereas phyllodes tumors often have an infiltrative or indistinct edge. Mitoses are very infrequent in fibroadenoma, and stromal cells usually have minimal pleomorphism.

Several important points should be noted in distinguishing phyllodes tumor from fibroadenoma:

1. The exact threshold for degree of stromal cellularity in distinguishing a cellular fibroadenoma from benign phyllodes tumor is not clearly defined, and distinction between these lesions should be based on a constellation of histologic features.

△△	*Differential Diagnosis* PHYLLODES TUMOR

- Versus benign or borderline phyllodes tumor:
- Cellular fibroadenoma
- Versus malignant phyllodes tumor
- Sarcomatoid metaplastic carcinoma
- Sarcoma—primary or metastatic

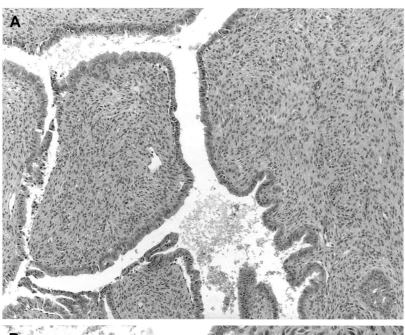

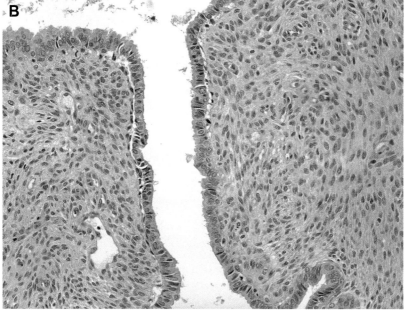

Fig. 2. Phyllodes tumor. (*A*) At low power (×40), note the leaflike projections of cellular stroma surfaced by epithelium that protrude into cyst. (*B*) At higher power (×200), note the cellular stroma. (This tumor was categorized as benign.)

2. A prominent intracanalicular (leaflike) pattern does not automatically equate with a diagnosis of phyllodes tumor in the absence of other characteristics (such as cellular stroma). In phyllodes tumor, the fronds of cellular stroma, which are covered by epithelium, project into cystic spaces and usually do not conform exactly to the shape of the cysts into which they project. In contrast, a predominantly intracanalicular pattern in fibroadenoma (even if leaflike) tends to be more compressed, with fronds conforming to the potential spaces into which they project (akin to an orderly, well-fitting jigsaw puzzle).

3. Lack of a prominent leaflike growth pattern in a lesion with cellular stroma does not preclude a diagnosis of phyllodes tumor. Cellular fibroadenoma tends to have a more uniform, orderly architectural pattern at low power, with a microscopically well-circumscribed edge. In contrast, phyllodes tumors tend to be more

Fig. 3. Phyllodes tumor. (*A*) At low power (×20), the tumor edge is infiltrative. (*B*) At intermediate power (×100), the cellular stroma can easily be seen. (*C*) At higher power (×200), the stroma is markedly cellular, with stromal cell pleomorphism and easily identified mitotic figures. (This tumor was categorized as malignant.)

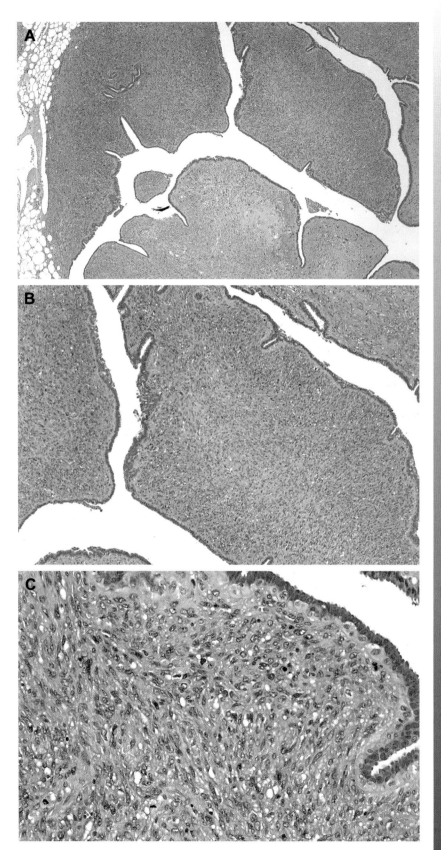

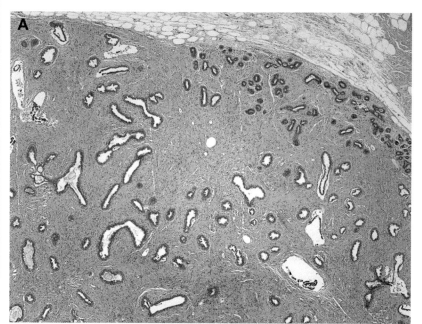

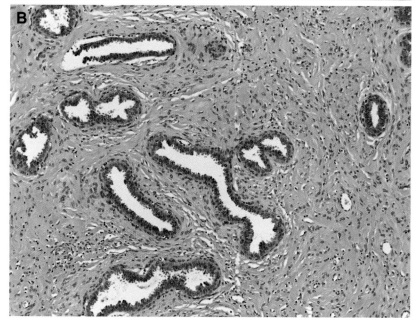

Fig. 4. Cellular stroma. (*A*) The tumor has a well-circumscribed border and an orderly pericanalicular growth pattern at low power (×40). (*B*) At higher power (×200), the mildly increased stromal cellularity, with bland-appearing stromal cells, is demonstrated.

heterogeneous in stromal cellularity and in arrangement of glands and stroma.

4. The stroma in phyllodes tumors may be less cellular in areas; however, this does not negate the diagnosis when other classic features are present (**Fig. 5**). Phyllodes tumors may have areas that resemble fibroadenomas and should therefore be well sampled. As alluded, phyllodes tumors tend to be more heterogeneous in stromal cellularity than fibroadenomas. A helpful distinguishing feature, if present, is enhancement of stromal cellularity in the zone adjacent to the epithelium in phyllodes tumor ("periductal condensation of stroma").

5. Stromal mitoses may also be seen in fibroadenomas (up to 2 per 10 high power fields) and, in the absence of diagnostic features of phyllodes tumor, should not be used solely to diagnose

Fig. 5. Phyllodes tumor with variably cellular stroma. (*A*) At scanning power (×20), note the enhanced intracanalicular leaflike growth pattern and infiltrative edge. (*B*) At intermediate power (×100), note the variability in stromal cellularity. (*C*) Stroma is often most cellular in the subepithelial zone, seen at high power (×200).

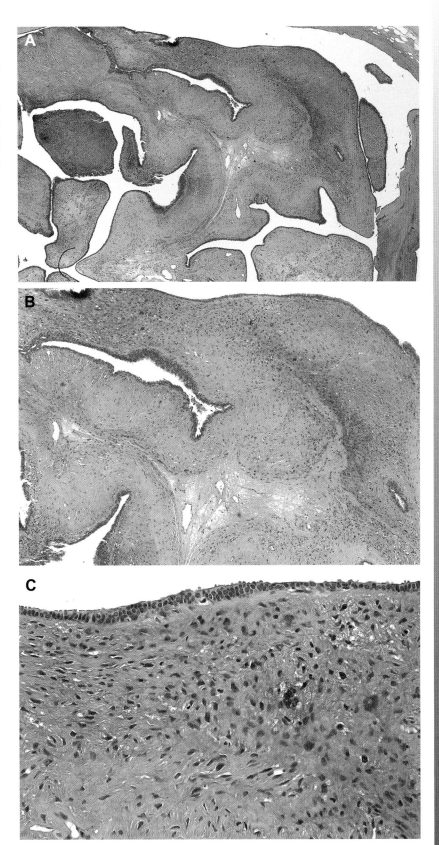

the latter. Stromal mitoses, however, are more often seen in the subepithelial zone.

6. Phyllodes tumors often demonstrate an infiltrative tumor edge. Although this edge may take the form of tongues of stroma infiltrating into adjacent breast parenchyma, it more often consists of an irregular interface with surrounding adipose tissue, with interposed lesional stromal cells.

7. The presence of multinucleated stromal giant cells in an otherwise classic fibroadenoma does not negate that diagnosis.[23,24] Microscopically, these giant cells are similar to those found at other sites (such as the lower female genital tract, nasal polyps, anus, and bladder) and are cells with multiple hyperchromatic nuclei grouped in tight clusters, frequently forming wreathlike (floret) patterns. This close arrangement of several smaller cells with minimal cytoplasm may be confused with one larger cell on low- or intermediatepower examination. An important clue to their benignity is that these multinucleated stromal giant cells appear "out of phase" with the other stromal cells present, which have bland cytologic features without pleomorphism, increased cellularity, or mitotic activity.

It is unfortunate that due to overlapping features, some cellular fibroepithelial lesions may defy definitive categorization as cellular fibroadenoma or as benign phyllodes tumor. A conservative approach is prudent in such cases, particularly when the lesion is adjacent to a surgical resection margin and it is unclear whether transection has occurred. A diagnosis of FELCS, with a comment communicating the difficulty in categorization, a description of the features, and a suggestion to consider re-excision if the lesion appears to be transected, may be the best approach in such circumstances.

Malignant phyllodes tumors should be distinguished from frankly malignant spindle cell tumors such as sarcomatoid or spindle cell metaplastic carcinomas, or more rarely sarcomas (metastatic or primary). Adequate sampling of a lesion that appears to be a sarcoma of the breast is very important, with careful microscopic examination to exclude a phyllodes tumor that has marked stromal overgrowth and a minimal epithelial component. Often only one histologic section may show a focal slitlike epithelial component. In addition to thorough hematoxylin and eosin microscopy, immunohistochemistry may be helpful, particularly in distinguishing a metaplastic carcinoma (ie, immunostaining spindle cells with high molecular weight cytokeratins and p63).

DIAGNOSIS

In an attempt to predict clinical behavior (ie, chance of local recurrence or distant metastasis), several classification schemes have been proposed for phyllodes tumors, including two- and three-tier systems.[14,25–27] One two-tier system includes "low-grade" and "high-grade" categories;[26] however, this system is problematic due to its malignant connotation, particularly with respect to otherwise benign "low-grade" lesions that have minimal chance of metastasis. A more clinically relevant scheme is a three-tier system that categorizes phyllodes tumors as "benign," "borderline," and "malignant."[13–15] This categorization is based on semiquantitatively applying several histologic features, an approach originally effectively proposed by Norris and Taylor[28] and later used by Pietrushka and Barnes,[29] Hart and colleagues,[30] and Ward and Evans.[31]

The histologic features used in this three-tier system include the following:

Degree of stromal cellularity
Degree of stromal cell pleomorphism
Stromal mitotic count
Tumor border (ie, circumscribed or invasive)
Presence of stromal overgrowth, as originally described as a low power microscopic field ($\times$40 total = $\times$4 objective and $\times$10 ocular) with stroma but no epithelium[30,31]
Presence of heterologous sarcomatous elements (ie, other than fibrosarcoma; eg, liposarcoma, osteosarcoma, chondrosarcoma), automatically qualifying a phyllodes tumor as malignant (**Fig. 6**)[28,31–34]

This latter finding is the strongest to be associated with metastasis in a malignant phyllodes tumor. Therefore, multiple sections should be taken and sections should be carefully scrutinized to avoid missing focal heterologous elements. The presence of benign heterologous mesenchymal elements (such as chondroid and lipomatous areas), however, does not automatically qualify a lesion as malignant in the absence of other features.[35,36]

Benign phyllodes tumors have moderately increased stromal cellularity, little stromal cell pleomorphism, few mitoses (<5 per 10 high power fields), and a generally well-circumscribed, pushing margin. Stromal overgrowth is rare, and heterologous sarcomatous elements are not found. In contrast, malignant phyllodes tumors have markedly cellular stroma, marked stromal cell pleomorphism, and abundant easily identified mitoses (>10 per 10 high power fields). Margins

Fig. 6. Malignant phyllodes tumor with liposarcomatous heterologous elements. (*A*) At low power (×40), note the retained leaflike enhanced intracanalicular pattern. (*B*) Lipoblasts are demonstrated at high power (×400).

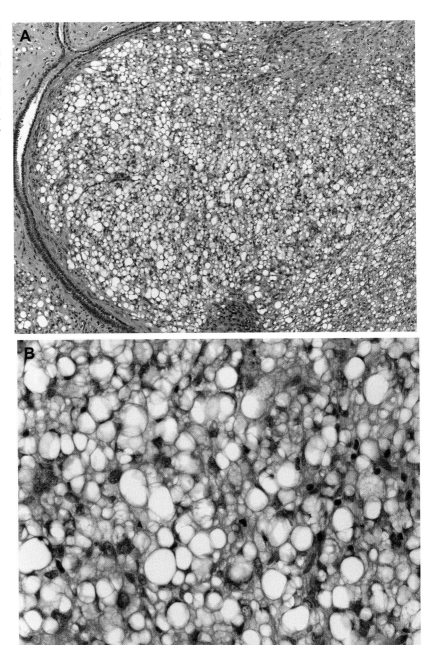

are invasive and stromal overgrowth is present. Heterologous sarcomatous elements may be found. (In other words, malignant phyllodes tumors are frankly high-grade and would be considered high-grade sarcomas in any other site in the body). Borderline phyllodes tumors have features between these two extremes—not frankly malignant but one or two worrisome features such as stromal overgrowth or 5 to 10 mitoses per 10 high power fields. Not uncommonly, the distinction between benign and borderline phyllodes tumor may be gray. In such cases, rather than trying to shoehorn the case into a benign or borderline diagnostic category, a more prudent approach would be a top-line diagnosis of phyllodes tumor, with a note describing the features present and proximity to resection margins, and a comment that the lesion has a high likelihood of recurrence if incompletely excised but a very low probability of metastasis.

As with phyllodes tumors in general, the incidence of benign, borderline, and malignant phyllodes tumors varies by population studied (ie, tertiary referral center versus community setting). In addition, the reported incidence of malignant phyllodes tumors varies by histologic criteria used.[37] In general, the overall frequency of malignant phyllodes tumors appears to be below 20%;[13] however, the true incidence of frankly malignant phyllodes tumors with metastatic potential is probably far lower—in the single-digit percentages.[37] This paucity of malignant tumors among an already uncommon tumor limits the power of clinical studies to determine robust predictors of outcome.

PROGNOSIS

Local recurrence of phyllodes tumors occurs irrespective of histologic category (ie, benign, borderline, or malignant) and is most strongly associated with adequacy of surgical excision (**Fig. 7**).[14,27,36,38–46] For example, in one community-based study of 32 phyllodes tumors (Nottingham),[14] all seven recurrences had positive margins on initial surgical excision (including 6 of 23 benign phyllodes tumors and 1 of 5 malignant tumors). In contrast, there were no recurrences among tumors excised with negative margins (10 benign tumors and all 4 borderline tumors). In a retrospective 40-year study at a large tertiary referral center

(Memorial Sloan Kettering),[47] 28 of 150 benign phyllodes tumors and 4 of 49 malignant phyllodes tumors recurred, most of which were incompletely excised. The average time to recurrence in this study was 2 years; however, in some cases, many years elapsed (up to 28). Although it should be strongly reiterated that phyllodes tumors, regardless of histologic category, require adequate excision, the exact extent of the negative margin required is not known. Of importance, there appears to be no difference in survival for patients who have malignant phyllodes tumor based on surgical treatment (ie, local versus mastectomy),[12,43] and furthermore, adjuvant radiation therapy appears to play no role.[12] In contrast to most reports emphasizing the importance of clear margins, a few investigators have advocated a "wait and see" policy for phyllodes tumors found unexpectedly without initial wide resection.[48] Close clinical and imaging follow-up would be needed in this situation,[49] and this approach is not generally recommended.

Older reports assumed that local recurrence was a sign of malignancy in phyllodes tumors,[50,51] but as previously noted, recurrence occurs irrespective of histologic category (ie, benign, borderline, or malignant). In fact, most patients who develop a recurrence do not develop distant metastases (a defining feature of malignancy).[14,47] The overall rate of metastasis from phyllodes tumors is low at 10% or less, and even histologically malignant phyllodes tumors metastasize in 22% or fewer cases and borderline tumors in 4%

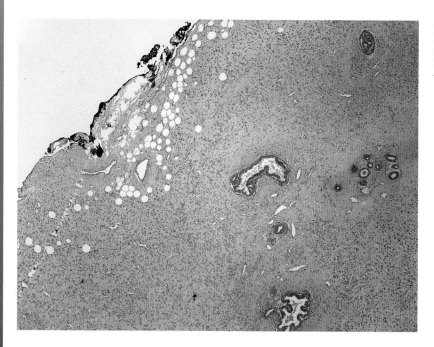

Fig. 7. Borderline phyllodes tumor at inked resection margin. Note infiltration of adipose tissue (×100).

or fewer. Some investigators have reported that tumors carefully categorized as borderline do not metastasize.[43] Malignant phyllodes tumors usually metastasize in a sarcomatous pattern, with the spindle cell component involving lungs, pleura, and bone.[12,41,52,53] Very rarely, a metastasis may be composed of stromal and epithelial components.[54] Axillary metastases are extremely rare; therefore, axillary lymph node sampling is not indicated and does not alter survival.[55] The best predictors of distant metastases are the presence of truly sarcomatous elements (particularly those that are heterologous)[28,29,31–34] and stromal overgrowth.[31,34] Indeed, metastases are extremely unlikely without these features. Other features, such as tumor necrosis, do not appear to be independent predictors of metastasis. In an excellent recent review, Carter and Page[49] called into question the utility of a "borderline category," considering that these lesions have such a low chance of metastasis and their recurrence rate is similar to benign tumors when adequately excised. Philosophically, these investigators suggested that efforts should be directed to the identification of a purely malignant category that would predict the potential to metastasize.[49] A primary reason for the borderline category may be to prevent overdiagnosis of malignancy in patients not overtly at risk of metastasis.[49]

Several recent studies have used a variety of immunohistochemical markers in an attempt to predict clinical outcome of phyllodes tumors; however, results have been disappointing. Although most markers have correlated well with histologic category or grade of phyllodes tumors, most have not been shown to independently predict outcome (ie, local recurrence or metastases).

Proliferation by Ki-67 (MIB1) immunostaining has been used by several investigators.[16,27,56–61] For example, Kleer and colleagues[27] demonstrated good correlation between Ki-67 labeling and histologic grade of phyllodes tumors, but it was not an independent predictor of risk of metastasis or local recurrence. Similarly, Kocova and colleagues[56] and Umekita and Yoshida[58] demonstrated good correlation of MIB1 index with the histologic category of phyllodes tumor but not as an independent predictor of outcome. Of interest, Shpitz and colleagues[60] showed that progression to a more malignant morphology in recurrences was accompanied by a higher proliferation rate by Ki-67 immunostaining.

Staining for p53 has also been used in an attempt to categorize phyllodes tumors.[16,27,57,59,60,62–67] In one study, Feakins and colleagues[63] reported good correlation between histologic parameters (eg, stromal nuclear pleomorphism, mitotic count, stromal overgrowth, infiltrative margin) and p53 stromal expression, but as with Ki-67, this correlation did not predict for tumor recurrence or survival. Similar results have been reported by Tse and colleagues[65,66] and by Tan and colleagues.[67] Shpitz and colleagues[60] did not find that p53 predicted recurrence but reported more immunostaining in tumors with "more malignant potential."

CD117 (c-Kit) immunostaining has also been tested in phyllodes tumors with a view to predict clinical outcome and as a potential therapeutic target.[67–70] Chen and colleagues[68] correlated expression of CD117, CD34, and actin with histologic grade of 19 phyllodes tumors. They reported expression of CD34 more often in benign tumors, whereas CD117 and actin were more often found in histologically malignant tumors, but these findings were not independently related to clinical outcome. Similarly, Tse and colleagues[69] reported a strong correlation between CD117 immunostaining and increasing histologic grade (ie, malignant > borderline > benign); however, findings were not related to outcome. In a recent tissue microarray-based study, Tan and colleagues[67] reported strong correlation of stromal CD117 immunostaining with histologic category/grade. Of interest, stromal CD117 positivity was also more likely in patients who had tumors that recurred (7/31 [23%]) compared with tumors that did not (10/242 [4%]) using univariate analysis but was not tested for independence among other parameters such as histologic grade or margin status.

Other markers studied also have not independently predicted outcome and include platelet-derived growth factor,[71] vascular endothelial growth factor,[72] estrogen and progesterone receptor in the epithelial component,[73] HER2,[60] and epidermal growth factor receptor.[74]

Lae and colleagues[75] recently compared comparative genomic hybridization data with histologic categorization in 30 phyllodes tumors. Recurrent chromosome imbalances were observed in 55% of benign, 91% of borderline, and 100% of malignant phyllodes tumors. Mean chromosome changes included 1 in the benign category versus 6 in each of the borderline and malignant categories. Gains of 1q were found in only 1 of 9 benign tumors but were found in 11 of 21 borderline or malignant tumors. These investigators concluded that there were two distinct patterns of genomic imbalance in phyllodes tumors that could distinguish between histologically benign lesions (with none or a few chromosome changes) and borderline or malignant lesions (with numerous recurrent chromosomal changes, in particular 1q gain and 13q loss).[75]

CELLULAR FIBROEPITHELIAL LESIONS ON CORE BIOPSY

DIAGNOSTIC ALGORITHM

A diagnosis of fibroadenoma can usually be readily made based on histologic features seen on core needle biopsy (CNB) specimens (**Fig. 8**). Therefore, when diagnosed on CNB, these lesions can be safely managed by observation alone, provided that the imaging studies are concordant with that diagnosis and there are no other lesions for which an excision would be indicated (such as atypical ductal hyperplasia). In contrast, the differential diagnosis of FELCS on CNB ranges from cellular fibroadenoma to phyllodes tumor (**Fig. 9**). (These diagnostic dilemmas, of course, do not include markedly cellular and pleomorphic spindle cell lesions on CNB, in which the diagnosis of malignancy is not at issue, but rather the differential diagnosis is between malignant phyllodes tumor, metaplastic carcinoma, and high-grade sarcoma.) Until more recently, the few follow-up studies of cellular fibroepithelial lesions on CNB had small patient numbers, with limited pathologic details on CNB or excision specimens, and included mostly reviews of pathology reports rather than detailed reviews of slides by the study pathologists.[76–79]

Seattle and Nottingham Studies

Two recent studies have had larger patient cohorts, and the study pathologists evaluated in detail the pathologic features of CNB specimens with the aim of elucidating features useful in predicting the probability of phyllodes tumor occurring rather than fibroadenoma.[16,80] In one study, Jacobs and colleagues (Seattle, Washington)[16] identified 29 consecutive cases of FELCS on CNB from their files and correlated the pathologic features of CNB specimens with outcome on subsequent surgical excision (and with clinical and imaging data). In contrast, a second study by Lee and colleagues (Nottingham, UK)[80] used a slightly different approach, starting with the diagnosis made on surgical excision (36 phyllodes tumors and 38 fibroadenomas) and then correlating these diagnoses with histologic features of the preceding CNB specimens.

Seattle study

In the Seattle study, all 29 patients who had FELCS on CNB had excision follow-up as part of their routine care, resulting in 12 patients who had phyllodes tumors (5 benign, 6 borderline, 1 malignant) and 16 patients who had fibroadenomas (1 patient did not have a fibroepithelial lesion on excision).[16] The histologic features evaluated were selected to include those that had been reported to be of potential use in the pathologic categorization of phyllodes tumors, the prediction of clinical outcome, and the distinction from fibroadenoma (ie, stromal cellularity, stromal cell nuclear atypia, stromal mitoses, proportion of stroma to epithelium and stromal overgrowth, presence of an infiltrative edge, and predominant growth pattern).

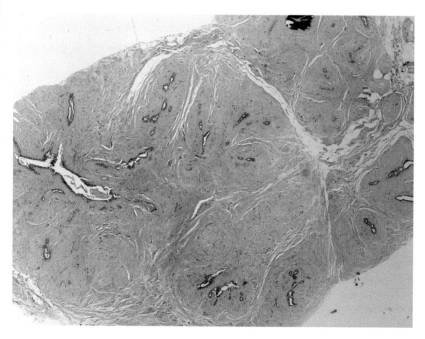

Fig. 8. Fibroadenoma on CNB ($\times$100).

Fig. 9. FELCS on CNB. This patient had a phyllodes tumor at surgical excision. (*A*) ×40. (*B*) ×400.

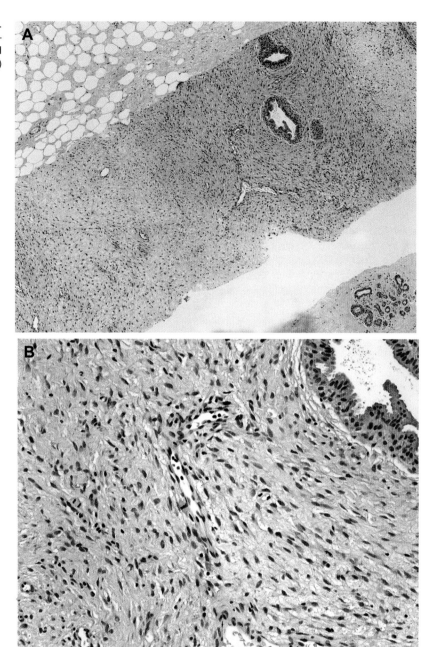

CNB specimens were also immunostained for the proliferation markers Ki-67 and topoisomerase 2α and for p53, on the basis of reports of their use in categorizing phyllodes tumors and their distinction from fibroadenoma. In addition, imaging and clinical findings were correlated with excision outcome. Among the histologic parameters, only stromal cellularity (markedly increased versus mildly increased) and presence of stromal mitoses were independently predictive of the presence of phyllodes tumor versus fibroadenoma at excision. Proliferation indices by immunohistochemistry (Ki67 and topoisomerase 2α) were significantly different among FELCS on CNB, which resulted in phyllodes tumor versus those that resulted in fibroadenoma at excision.[16] Although significant in multivariate analysis, there was overlap between categories, limiting the clinical value of proliferation markers in individual patients. Immunostaining for p53 was not a helpful predictor.

Nottingham study

In the Nottingham study,[80] the 36 phyllodes tumor excisions were preceded by 44 CNBs, and the 38 fibroadenomas were preceded by 37 CNBs. The features most likely to be found in a fibroepithelial lesion on CNB that preceded a diagnosis of phyllodes tumor rather than fibroadenoma included increased stromal cellularity and, in contrast to the study by the Seattle group (likely due to the use of smaller than traditional microscopic field sizes by Lee and colleagues[80]), stromal overgrowth, fragmentation of cores, and adipose tissue interposed with stroma.[80] Although both studies reported that growth pattern (in particular a leaflike morphology) was not useful on core biopsy, the Nottingham study found that fragmentation of cores was a useful feature predictive of phyllodes tumor at excision. This fragmentation or cores is probably due to the enhanced intracanalicular and cystic pattern present in phyllodes tumors, resulting in discontinuous tissue cores traversing these spaces. The Seattle group found an infiltrative edge in 36% of the CNB specimens that resulted in fibroadenoma and in 63% of those that resulted in phyllodes tumor (although this difference was not statistically significant), whereas the Nottingham group found poor interobserver variability with this feature. The Nottingham pathologists found that the presence of adipose tissue interposed with stroma was a more useful surrogate and helpful for predicting phyllodes tumor at excision. It should be noted, however, that otherwise classic fibroadenomas may contain foci of benign adipose tissue, calling into question the predictive value of this feature.

Although the Seattle and Nottingham studies differ in design, they both highlight the limitations of CNB (which is essentially a sampling procedure) and the difficulty of extrapolating histologic criteria that are useful for excision specimens to the context of CNB specimens. For example, the Seattle group[16] found that an enhanced intracanalicular leaflike pattern, an invasive lesional border, and stromal overgrowth at ×40 total power (which are all useful for diagnosing phyllodes tumors in surgical excision specimens) were unhelpful in discriminating between FELCS in CNB specimens. In addition, some phyllodes tumors might have areas with relatively less stromal cellularity that are similar in appearance to fibroadenoma and would therefore be subject to sampling issues by CNB. A theoretic concern is for a false-negative CNB diagnosis (ie, a fibroadenoma on CNB when the targeted lesion is a phyllodes tumor),

particularly in larger lesions due intratumoral heterogeneity or in a phyllodes tumor arising in fibroadenoma;[81] however, the estimated true false-negative rate has been reported to be lower than 1%.[80]

Recommendations for core needle biopsy and excision

Based on the significant probability of phyllodes tumor occurring in patients who have cellular fibroepithelial lesions diagnosed on CNB (up to 41% in the Seattle study, which was the largest study to specifically examine outcome of CNBs with a diagnosis of FELCS), it remains prudent for patients diagnosed with FELCS on CNB to undergo surgical excision; however, the optimal surgical management differs for phyllodes tumors compared with fibroadenomas (ie, negative margins versus enucleation of the lesion, respectively.) Treating all patients who have FELCS on CNB with the same surgical procedure might, depending on the quantity of tissue removed, result in excessive surgery for patients who have fibroadenomas or result in insufficient surgery for patients who have phyllodes tumors. In addition, achieving negative margins at the time of primary excision for phyllodes tumor is preferable to re-excision that would likely involve removal of more tissue and less favorable cosmetic results.

Radiologic features

In keeping with prior reports, the Seattle group demonstrated that radiologic features[17–19] and clinical parameters such as patient age and tumor size were not useful in predicting the presence of phyllodes tumor at excision.[16] Perhaps assessment of velocity of growth by imaging might be a more useful guide.[82]

Surgical treatment

The pathologic features gleaned from the Seattle and Nottingham studies may help guide surgical treatment. For example, the Seattle group suggested combining the degree of stromal cellularity, mitoses, and proliferation indices in CNB specimens to assess the probability of a FELCS being a fibroadenoma or phyllodes tumor and, therefore, guiding management of these lesions.[16] These investigators suggest the following probabilistic model:

> FELCS in CNB specimens that have markedly increased stromal cellularity or those with moderately increased stromal cellularity, stromal mitoses, and elevated proliferation marker indices have the highest probability of being phyllodes tumors.

Pitfalls

! Phyllodes tumors may be smaller and may occur in younger patients—size and age are not discriminatory versus fibroadenoma.

! Stromal cellularity may be variable, with some areas of phyllodes tumor resembling fibroadenoma. Extensive sampling is advised to avoid underdiagnosis.

! Malignant phyllodes tumors often exhibit marked stromal overgrowth. Incomplete pathologic sampling may result in missing the epithelial component and a misdiagnosis as sarcoma.

Those with moderately increased stromal cellularity, no stromal mitoses, and low proliferation marker indices might be fibroadenomas or phyllodes tumors.

Those with mildly increased stromal cellularity, especially those with no mitoses and low proliferation indices, are more likely to be fibroadenomas.

Further prospective clinical outcome studies may assist in further refining probabilistic approaches such as those proposed by Jacobs and colleagues.[16]

Based on the inherent variability in CNB sampling, the low predictive power of imaging, and the subjective nature of the assessment of certain pathologic features of CNB specimens (in particular the degree of stromal cellularity), it remains prudent that all patients who have FELCS diagnosed on CNB should undergo surgical excision.

REFERENCES

1. Lerwill MF. Biphasic lesions of the breast. Semin Diagn Pathol 2004;21(1):48–56.

2. Dupont WD, Page DL, Parl FF, et al. Long-term risk of breast cancer in women with fibroadenoma. N Engl J Med 1994;331(1):10–5.

3. Sklair-Levy M, Sella T, Alweiss T, et al. Incidence and management of complex fibroadenomas. AJR Am J Roentgenol 2008;190(1):214–8.

4. Oberman HA. Breast lesions in the adolescent female. In: Sommers SC, Rosen PP, editors. Pathology Annual, Part 1. Norwalk (CT): Appleton-Century-Crofts; 1979.

5. Nambiar R, Kutty MK. Giant fibro-adenoma (cystosarcoma phyllodes) in adolescent females—a clinicopathological study. Br J Surg 1974;61(2):113–7.

6. Ashikari R, Farrow JH, O'Hara J. Fibroadenomas in the breast of juveniles. Surg Gynecol Obstet 1971; 132(2):259–62.

7. Mies C, Rosen PP. Juvenile fibroadenoma with atypical epithelial hyperplasia. Am J Surg Pathol 1987; 11(3):184–90.

8. Dyer NH, Bridger JE, Taylor RS. Cystosarcoma phylloides. Br J Surg 1966;53(5):450–5.

9. Kessinger A, Foley JF, Lemon HM, et al. Metastatic cystosarcoma phyllodes: a case report and review of the literature. J Surg Oncol 1972;4(2):131–47.

10. Keelan PA, Myers JL, Wold LE, et al. Phyllodes tumor: clinicopathologic review of 60 patients and flow cytometric analysis in 30 patients. Hum Pathol 1992;23(9):1048–54.

11. Rajan PB, Cranor ML, Rosen PP. Cystosarcoma phyllodes in adolescent girls and young women: a study of 45 patients. Am J Surg Pathol 1998; 22(1):64–9.

12. Chaney AW, Pollack A, McNeese MD, et al. Primary treatment of cystosarcoma phyllodes of the breast. Cancer 2000;89(7):1502–11.

13. Tavassoli FA, Devilee P. Pathology and genetics: tumours of the breast and female genital organs. In: Kleihues P, Sobin LH, editors. World Health Organization classification of tumours. Lyon (France): IARC Press; 2003. p. 99–103.

14. Moffat CJ, Pinder SE, Dixon AR, et al. Phyllodes tumours of the breast: a clinicopathological review of thirty-two cases. Histopathology 1995;27(3): 205–18.

15. Elston CW, Ellis IO, Fibroadenoma and related conditions. In: Elston CW, Ellis IO, editors. The breast, vol. 13. 3rd edition. Edinburgh (UK): Churchill Livingstone; 1998. p. 147–86

16. Jacobs TW, Chen YY, Guinee DG Jr, et al. Fibroepithelial lesions with cellular stroma on breast core needle biopsy: are there predictors of outcome on surgical excision? Am J Clin Pathol 2005;124(3): 342–54.

17. Buchberger W, Strasser K, Heim K, et al. Phylloides tumor: findings on mammography, sonography, and aspiration cytology in 10 cases. AJR Am J Roentgenol 1991;157(4):715–9.

18. Cosmacini P, Zurrida S, Veronesi P, et al. Phyllode tumor of the breast: mammographic experience in 99 cases. Eur J Radiol 1992;15(1):11–4.

19. Liberman L, Bonaccio E, Hamele-Bena D, et al. Benign and malignant phyllodes tumors: mammographic and sonographic findings. Radiology 1996;198(1):121–4.

20. Yilmaz E, Sal S, Lebe B. Differentiation of phyllodes tumors versus fibroadenomas. Acta Radiol 2002; 43(1):34–9.

21. Chao TC, Lo YF, Chen SC, et al. Sonographic features of phyllodes tumors of the breast. Ultrasound Obstet Gynecol 2002;20(1):64–71.

22. Rosen PP. Rosen's breast pathology. 2nd edition. Philadelphia: Lippincott-Raven; 2001.

23. Berean K, Tron VA, Churg A, et al. Mammary fibroadenoma with multinucleated stromal giant cells. Am J Surg Pathol 1986;10(11):823–7.

24. Powell CM, Cranor ML, Rosen PP. Multinucleated stromal giant cells in mammary fibroepithelial neoplasms. A study of 11 patients. Arch Pathol Lab Med 1994;118(9):912–6.

25. Layfield LJ, Hart J, Neuwirth H, et al. Relation between DNA ploidy and the clinical behavior of phyllodes tumors. Cancer 1989;64(7):1486–9.

26. Tavassoli FA. Pathology of the breast. 2nd edition. Stamford (CT): Appleton and Lange; 1999.

27. Kleer CG, Giordano TJ, Braun T, et al. Pathologic, immunohistochemical, and molecular features of benign and malignant phyllodes tumors of the breast. Mod Pathol 2001;14(3):185–90.

28. Norris HJ, Taylor HB. Relationship of histologic features to behavior of cystosarcoma phyllodes. Analysis of ninety-four cases. Cancer 1967;20(12):2090–9.

29. Pietruszka M, Barnes L. Cystosarcoma phyllodes: a clinicopathologic analysis of 42 cases. Cancer 1978;41(5):1974–83.

30. Hart WR, Bauer RC, Oberman HA. Cystosarcoma phyllodes. A clinicopathologic study of twenty-six hypercellular periductal stromal tumors of the breast. Am J Clin Pathol 1978;70(2):211–6.

31. Ward RM, Evans HL. Cystosarcoma phyllodes. A clinicopathologic study of 26 cases. Cancer 1986;58(10):2282–9.

32. Qizilbash AH. Cystosarcoma phyllodes with liposarcomatous stroma. Am J Clin Pathol 1976;65(3):321–7.

33. Cohn-Cedermark G, Rutqvist LE, Rosendahl I, et al. Prognostic factors in cystosarcoma phyllodes. A clinicopathologic study of 77 patients. Cancer 1991;68(9):2017–22.

34. Hawkins RE, Schofield JB, Fisher C, et al. The clinical and histologic criteria that predict metastases from cystosarcoma phyllodes. Cancer 1992;69(1):141–7.

35. Powell CM, Rosen PP. Adipose differentiation in cystosarcoma phyllodes. A study of 14 cases. Am J Surg Pathol 1994;18(7):720–7.

36. Tan PH, Jayabaskar T, Chuah KL, et al. Phyllodes tumors of the breast: the role of pathologic parameters. Am J Clin Pathol 2005;123(4):529–40.

37. Parker SJ, Harries SA. Phyllodes tumours. Postgrad Med J 2001;77(909):428–35.

38. Hart J, Layfield LJ, Trumbull WE, et al. Practical aspects in the diagnosis and management of cystosarcoma phyllodes. Arch Surg 1988;123(9):1079–83.

39. Salvadori B, Cusumano F, Del Bo R, et al. Surgical treatment of phyllodes tumors of the breast. Cancer 1989;63(12):2532–6.

40. McGregor GI, Knowling MA, Este FA. Sarcoma and cystosarcoma phyllodes tumors of the breast—a retrospective review of 58 cases. Am J Surg 1994;167(5):477–80.

41. Reinfuss M, Mitus J, Duda K, et al. The treatment and prognosis of patients with phyllodes tumor of the breast: an analysis of 170 cases. Cancer 1996;77(5):910–6.

42. de Roos WK, Kaye P, Dent DM. Factors leading to local recurrence or death after surgical resection of phyllodes tumours of the breast. Br J Surg 1999;86(3):396–9.

43. Barth RJ Jr. Histologic features predict local recurrence after breast conserving therapy of phyllodes tumors. Breast Cancer Res Treat 1999;57(3):291–5.

44. Mangi AA, Smith BL, Gadd MA, et al. Surgical management of phyllodes tumors. Arch Surg 1999;134(5):487–92 [discussion: 492–83].

45. Chen WH, Cheng SP, Tzen CY, et al. Surgical treatment of phyllodes tumors of the breast: retrospective review of 172 cases. J Surg Oncol 2005;91(3):185–94.

46. Ben Hassouna J, Damak T, Gamoudi A, et al. Phyllodes tumors of the breast: a case series of 106 patients. Am J Surg 2006;192(2):141–7.

47. Hajdu SI, Espinosa MH, Robbins GF. Recurrent cystosarcoma phyllodes: a clinicopathologic study of 32 cases. Cancer 1976;38(3):1402–6.

48. Zurrida S, Bartoli C, Galimberti V, et al. Which therapy for unexpected phyllode tumour of the breast? Eur J Cancer 1992;28(2–3):654–7.

49. Carter BA, Page DL. Phyllodes tumor of the breast: local recurrence versus metastatic capacity. Hum Pathol 2004;35(9):1051–2.

50. Treves N, Sunderland DA. Cystosarcoma phyllodes of the breast: a malignant and a benign tumor; a clinicopathological study of seventy-seven cases. Cancer 1951;4(6):1286–332.

51. Lester J, Stout AP. Cystosarcoma phyllodes. Cancer 1954;7(2):335–53.

52. Kapiris I, Nasiri N, A'Hern R, et al. Outcome and predictive factors of local recurrence and distant metastases following primary surgical treatment of high-grade malignant phyllodes tumours of the breast. Eur J Surg Oncol 2001;27(8):723–30.

53. Asoglu O, Ugurlu MM, Blanchard K, et al. Risk factors for recurrence and death after primary surgical treatment of malignant phyllodes tumors. Ann Surg Oncol 2004;11(11):1011–7.

54. Kracht J, Sapino A, Bussolati G. Malignant phyllodes tumor of breast with lung metastases mimicking the primary. Am J Surg Pathol 1998;22(10):1284–90.

55. Geisler DP, Boyle MJ, Malnar KF, et al. Phyllodes tumors of the breast: a review of 32 cases. Am Surg 2000;66(4):360–6.

56. Kocova L, Skalova A, Fakan F, et al. Phyllodes tumour of the breast: immunohistochemical study

of 37 tumours using MIB1 antibody. Pathol Res Pract 1998;194(2):97–104.

57. Kuenen-Boumeester V, Henzen-Logmans SC, Timmermans MM, et al. Altered expression of p53 and its regulated proteins in phyllodes tumours of the breast. J Pathol 1999;189(2):169–75.

58. Umekita Y, Yoshida H. Immunohistochemical study of MIB1 expression in phyllodes tumor and fibroadenoma. Pathol Int 1999;49(9):807–10.

59. Niezabitowski A, Lackowska B, Rys J, et al. Prognostic evaluation of proliferative activity and DNA content in the phyllodes tumor of the breast: immunohistochemical and flow cytometric study of 118 cases. Breast Cancer Res Treat 2001;65(1):77–85.

60. Shpitz B, Bomstein Y, Sternberg A, et al. Immunoreactivity of p53, Ki-67, and c-erbB-2 in phyllodes tumors of the breast in correlation with clinical and morphologic features. J Surg Oncol 2002;79(2):86–92.

61. Ridgway PF, Jacklin RK, Ziprin P, et al. Perioperative diagnosis of cystosarcoma phyllodes of the breast may be enhanced by MIB-1 index. J Surg Res 2004;122(1):83–8.

62. Millar EK, Beretov J, Marr P, et al. Malignant phyllodes tumours of the breast display increased stromal p53 protein expression. Histopathology 1999;34(6):491–6.

63. Feakins RM, Mulcahy HE, Nickols CD, et al. p53 expression in phyllodes tumours is associated with histological features of malignancy but does not predict outcome. Histopathology 1999;35(2):162–9.

64. Gatalica Z, Finkelstein S, Lucio E, et al. p53 protein expression and gene mutation in phyllodes tumors of the breast. Pathol Res Pract 2001;197(3):183–7.

65. Tse GM, Putti TC, Kung FY, et al. Increased p53 protein expression in malignant mammary phyllodes tumors. Mod Pathol 2002;15(7):734–40.

66. Tse GM, Lui PC, Scolyer RA, et al. Tumour angiogenesis and p53 protein expression in mammary phyllodes tumors. Mod Pathol 2003;16(10):1007–13.

67. Tan PH, Jayabaskar T, Yip G, et al. p53 and c-kit (CD117) protein expression as prognostic indicators in breast phyllodes tumors: a tissue microarray study. Mod Pathol 2005;18(12):1527–34.

68. Chen CM, Chen CJ, Chang CL, et al. CD34, CD117, and actin expression in phyllodes tumor of the breast. J Surg Res 2000;94(2):84–91.

69. Tse GMK, Putti TC, Lui PC, et al. Increased c-kit (CD117) expression in malignant mammary phyllodes tumors. Mod Pathol 2004;17(7):827–31.

70. Koo CY, Bay BH, Lui PC, et al. Immunohistochemical expression of heparan sulfate correlates with stromal cell proliferation in breast phyllodes tumors. Mod Pathol 2006;19(10):1344–50.

71. Feakins RM, Wells CA, Young KA, et al. Platelet-derived growth factor expression in phyllodes tumors and fibroadenomas of the breast. Hum Pathol 2000; 31(10):1214–22.

72. Tse GM, Lui PC, Lee CS, et al. Stromal expression of vascular endothelial growth factor correlates with tumor grade and microvessel density in mammary phyllodes tumors: a multicenter study of 185 cases. Hum Pathol 2004;35(9):1053–7.

73. Tse GM, Lee CS, Kung FY, et al. Hormonal receptors expression in epithelial cells of mammary phyllodes tumors correlates with pathologic grade of the tumor: a multicenter study of 143 cases. Am J Clin Pathol 2002;118(4):522–6.

74. Tse GM, Lui PC, Vong JS, et al. Increased epidermal growth factor receptor (EGFR) expression in malignant mammary phyllodes tumors. Breast Cancer Res Treat 2008;11(3):441–8.

75. Lae M, Vincent-Salomon A, Savignoni A, et al. Phyllodes tumors of the breast segregate in two groups according to genetic criteria. Mod Pathol 2007;20(4):435–44.

76. Dershaw DD, Morris EA, Liberman L, et al. Nondiagnostic stereotaxic core breast biopsy: results of re-biopsy. Radiology 1996;198(2):323–5.

77. Meyer JE, Smith DN, Lester SC, et al. Large-needle core biopsy: nonmalignant breast abnormalities evaluated with surgical excision or repeat core biopsy. Radiology 1998;206(3):717–20.

78. Ioffe OB, Berg WA, Silverberg SG, et al. Mammographic-histopathologic correlation of large-core needle biopsies of the breast. Mod Pathol 1998; 11(8):721–7.

79. Komenaka IK, El-Tamer M, Pile-Spellman E, et al. Core needle biopsy as a diagnostic tool to differentiate phyllodes tumor from fibroadenoma. Arch Surg 2003;138(9):987–90.

80. Lee AH, Hodi Z, Ellis IO, et al. Histological features useful in the distinction of phyllodes tumour and fibroadenoma on needle core biopsy of the breast. Histopathology 2007;51(3):336–44.

81. Lee AH. Recent developments in the histological diagnosis of spindle cell carcinoma, fibromatosis and phyllodes tumour of the breast. Histopathology 2008;52(1):45–57.

82. Gordon PB, Gagnon FA, Lanzkowsky L. Solid breast masses diagnosed as fibroadenoma at fine-needle aspiration biopsy: acceptable rates of growth at long-term follow-up. Radiology 2003; 229(1):233–8.

ENCAPSULATED PAPILLARY CARCINOMA OF THE BREAST

Anna Marie Mulligan, MB, MSc, FRCPath

KEYWORDS

- Breast • Encapsulated papillary carcinoma • Intracystic papillary carcinoma
- Papillary lesions • Papilloma

ABSTRACT

Papillary lesions of the breast include a broad spectrum of entities, many of which can be diagnostically challenging for the pathologist. This article focuses on encapsulated papillary carcinoma, a recently proposed term used to describe papillary carcinoma occurring within a cystically dilated duct. Previously considered a variant of papillary ductal carcinoma in situ, the finding that these lesions typically lack myoepithelial cells at their periphery has raised questions about their true nature. This article presents a practical approach to the diagnosis of encapsulated papillary carcinoma with a review of its histologic mimics and clinical significance.

The term encapsulated papillary carcinoma recently was proposed by Hill and Yeh[1] to describe papillary carcinomas that are surrounded by a fibrous rim and lack evidence of stromal invasion. Rather than describing a new entity, this refers to a subset of lesions previously considered under the heading intracystic or encysted papillary carcinoma. These lesions generally have been considered to represent in situ processes; however, finding that at least a proportion lack myoepithelial cells at their periphery has called this view into question.

The proponents of the new terminology put forth the term encapsulated papillary carcinoma to reconcile the discrepancy in these in situ lesions that show absence of basal myoepithelial cell staining, suggesting that they represent part of a spectrum of progression intermediate between in situ and invasive carcinoma. In fact, that at least some of these lesions may represent invasive carcinomas has been suggested.[2] There is recognition that, whatever their true nature, their behavior is expected to be indolent with low metastatic potential.[3–5]

This article describes the morphologic features of encapsulated papillary carcinomas (EPCs) along with the various entities that may be considered in the differential diagnosis. A discussion on prognosis and management concludes the review. Of note, the descriptions and prognostic information are derived mostly from studies reported before the introduction of the new term.

Key Features
ENCAPSULATED PAPILLARY CARCINOMA

1. Describes a papillary carcinoma surrounded by a fibrotic rim without evidence of stromal invasion

2. Variably cystic and solid; solid growth may conceal papillary architecture

3. Arborizing fibrovascular cores lined by malignant epithelial cells without intervening myoepithelial cell layer

4. Epithelium proliferates between the fibrovascular cores to a varying degree, ranging from a single or several layers lining papillae to cribriform, solid, or micropapillary growth patterns

5. Usually low- or intermediate-grade, rarely high-grade with necrosis

6. Myoepithelial cells absent from periphery of lesion

Department of Laboratory Medicine, St. Michael's Hospital and University of Toronto, 30 Bond Street, Room 2-089 CCW, Toronto, Ontario M5B 1W8, Canada
E-mail address: mulligana@smh.toronto.on.ca

Surgical Pathology 2 (2009) 319–350
doi:10.1016/j.path.2009.02.008

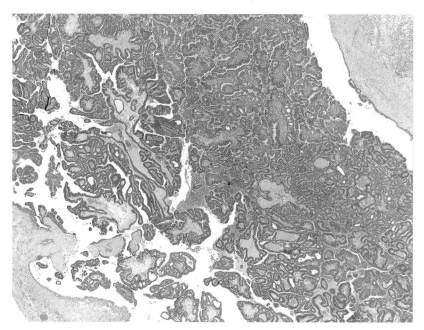

Fig. 1. Encapsulated papillary carcinoma (2.5 ×). Low-power view showing a cystically dilated duct with a fibrotic wall encircling the papillary growth.

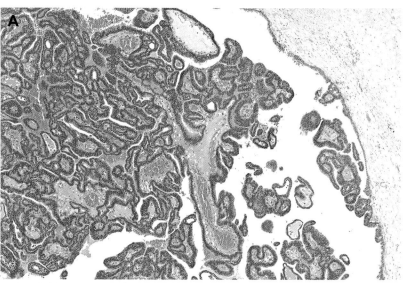

Fig. 2. (*A, B*) Encapsulated papillary carcinoma (5 × and 10 ×). An arborizing and complex papillary network lined by one or more layers of epithelium is seen. Note the uniformity of the cell population.

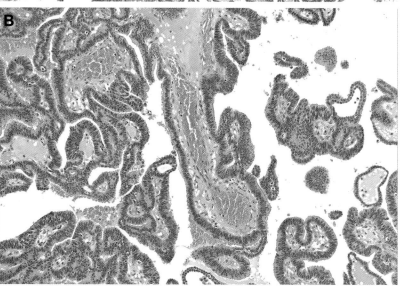

GROSS FEATURES

Lesions average 2 to 3 cm but can be significantly larger.[6] They are typically well-circumscribed with or without evidence of a fibrous capsule. The intracystic component varies in the proportion of solid and cystic elements and can be tan to red and hemorrhagic secondary to bleeding of the friable papillae. The consistency ranges from soft to firm if fibrosis is a prominent feature. Gross evidence of the papillary nature of the lesion will vary depending on the presence and extent of a solid component. Cystic lesions are more friable with detached papillary fragments and may be filled with partly clotted blood. The cyst wall is fibrotic and should be well-sampled to assess for stromal invasion.

MICROSCOPIC FEATURES

The designation of these lesions as intracystic was based on the belief that these tumors arose from the lining of breast cysts.[7,8] Although many do arise from larger more centrally placed ducts, it is probably the growth of the tumor and secretions that cause the cystic dilatation and eventual large size. The term EPC is reserved for those lesions that are solitary and discrete, typically involving large ducts.

The basic structure of a papillary lesion is the fibrovascular core. In cystic EPC, a dilated duct with a fibrotic wall encircles the papillary growth (**Fig. 1**). The latter shows an arborizing and complex papillary network lined by one or more layers of epithelium (**Fig. 2**). Cyst formation is not a prerequisite for the diagnosis, and, alternatively, a circumscribed solid nodule or nodules may be present (**Fig. 3**). In solid lesions, the papillary nature may be more difficult to appreciate given the compact nature of the tumor (**Fig. 4**). Carcinoma often extends into ducts at the periphery of the lesion. A key diagnostic feature is that the epithelium lies directly on the fibrovascular cores without an intervening myoepithelial cell layer (**Fig. 5**), although in a few cases, preservation of myoepithelial cells is at least focal.[9–11] Attention must be paid to the proliferating epithelium between the fibrovascular cores to distinguish benign from malignant lesions. The cytologic and architectural features will be those of other intraductal carcinomas, but with a papillary scaffold. The malignant epithelium can grow as a single layer lining the papillae (**Fig. 6**A); it can proliferate with the formation of cribriform (**Fig. 6**B) or trabecular structures, or it may form solid sheets (**Fig. 6**C). An intricate series of secondary and tertiary arborizing branches can fuse with the formation of complex patterns of glandular spaces and solid areas. Nonetheless, fibrovascular cores, albeit often inconspicuous, will be present. The epithelium in EPC consists of hyperchromatic nuclei that are often low- or intermediate-grade with a low mitotic index (**Fig. 7**). Rarely, they may be high-grade, and tumor necrosis may be prominent.[12]

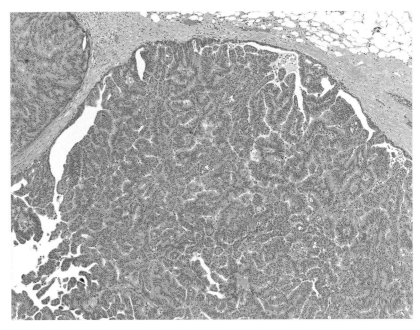

Fig. 3. Encapsulated papillary carcinoma (5 ×). Circumscribed nodules of tumor without cystic elements.

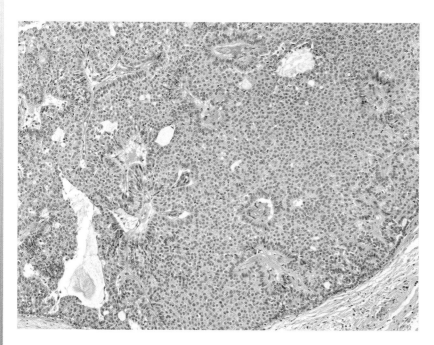

Fig. 4. Encapsulated papillary carcinoma (10 ×). The epithelium proliferates forming solid sheets, studded with fibrovascular cores. The compact growth of the epithelium can mask the papillary nature of the tumor.

MYOEPITHELIAL CELLS AND ENCAPSULATED PAPILLARY CARCINOMA

Although EPCs generally have been considered to represent in situ lesions, recent immunohistochemical studies have challenged this idea. Hill and Yeh[1] studied myoepithelial cell staining at the periphery of a range of papillary lesions using three specific and sensitive markers (calponin, smooth muscle myosin heavy chain, and p63). Absence or only focal staining of a basal myoepithelial cell layer was seen in five of nine cases of EPC. Intraluminal myoepithelial cells were not identified in any of these lesions. In contrast, all

25 benign intraductal papillomas (IPs) and all five cases of micropapillary ductal carcinoma in situ (DCIS) showed a distinct basal cell layer, and invasive papillary carcinomas showed virtually complete absence of staining. The cases lacking a basal myoepithelial cell layer consisted of large, expansile papillary lesions with pushing borders and fibrotic rims, prompting the authors to propose the term encapsulated papillary carcinoma, analogous to that seen in the thyroid.

This proposed change in terminology was consolidated further by findings from a subsequent study in which Collins and colleagues[2] used five myoepithelial cell markers (smooth muscle myosin heavy chain, calponin, p63, CD10, and CK 5/6) to evaluate the presence of myoepithelial cells at the periphery of a series of EPCs and IPs. In their 22 cases of EPC, myoepithelial cells were not identified at the periphery of the nodules with any of the five markers, nor were they identified histologically. This was in contrast to the continuous staining seen at the periphery of conventional DCIS and benign IP. As suggested by the authors, one explanation for this is that the myoepithelial cell layer has become markedly attenuated or altered because of their compression by the expansile growth of the lesion within the cystically dilated duct; however, in refute of this, all the IPs, including those with comparable sizes to the EPC, showed preservation of myoepithelial cell staining. An alternative explanation is that the nodules represent invasive, rather than in situ

---

△△ ***Differential Diagnosis***
ᴇɴᴄᴀᴘsᴜʟᴀᴛᴇᴅ Pᴀᴘɪʟʟᴀʀʏ Cᴀʀᴄɪɴᴏᴍᴀ

- Benign intraductal papilloma
- Atypical ductal hyperplasia (ADH) or DCIS arising within a benign intraductal papilloma
- Papillary ductal carcinoma in situ
- Solid papillary carcinoma
- Metastatic papillary carcinoma
- Carcinoma with cystic degeneration
- Invasive papillary carcinoma

Fig. *5.* Encapsulated papillary carcinoma (40 ×). The malignant epithelium lies directly on the fibrovascular cores without an intervening myoepithelial cell layer. Care must be taken not to overinterpret stromal fibroblasts and vascular endothelial cells within the fibrovascular cores as myoepithelial cells.

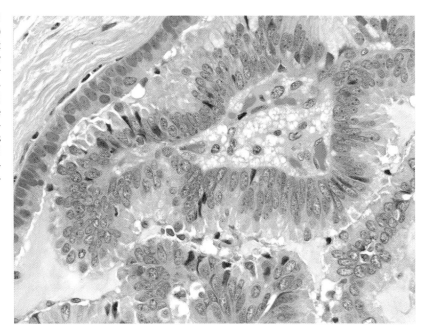

carcinoma, and although recent studies support an indolent course for these lesions,[3–5,13] as the authors point out, indolent behavior is not valid evidence that these are in situ lesions.

BENIGN INTRADUCTAL PAPILLOMA

Low-grade EPC may be difficult to differentiate from benign papillary lesions, the latter being far more common. These lesions consist of a papillary mass composed of branching fibrovascular cores within a cystically dilated duct (**Fig. 8**). The fibrovascular core forming the papillary structure is composed of a fibrous stalk with a centrally located vessel (**Fig. 9**). The core is lined by myoepithelial cells, and upon this layer, at least one layer of epithelium is found. The myoepithelial cells are usually round to cuboidal and often have clear cytoplasm (**Fig. 10**). The epithelial cells are usually columnar or cuboidal and have a lower nuclear-to-cytoplasmic ratio than the myoepithelial cells (**Fig. 11**). The epithelium may proliferate to greater or lesser degrees showing the characteristics seen with usual ductal hyperplasia (UDH) (**Fig. 12**). Important to note is that myoepithelial cells are typically absent from within the areas of hyperplasia, but, they will still be evident lining the fibrovascular cores upon which the epithelium is proliferating. Apocrine metaplasia of the epithelium is a not infrequent finding (**Fig. 13**). Squamous metaplasia can be seen but less frequently and usually following trauma. Occasionally the myoepithelial cells are prominent and show hyperplasia.

Conversely, they may be inconspicuous, and immunohistochemical markers may be necessary to identify them (**Fig. 14**).

Criteria for distinguishing benign from malignant papillary lesions were described by Kraus and Neubecker in 1962.[14] Although these criteria remain in use today, they are subject to numerous exceptions and structural variations,[15] contributing to the diagnostic challenge presented by papillary lesions. EPC and IP share many architectural features. The branching fibrovascular cores of the malignant lesion, however, are often less conspicuous and tend to be more delicate as opposed to the more fibrous-appearing cores of papillomas (**Fig. 15**). Fibrosis with epithelial entrapment within the fibrovascular cores is frequent in benign lesions. Benign apocrine metaplasia is not a feature of EPC, although apocrine differentiation can be seen (**Fig. 16**), the latter exhibiting cytologic atypia consistent with the rest of the tumor and in contrast to the bland foci of apocrine change encountered in IP. As discussed previously, myoepithelial cells are generally absent in EPC, in contrast to the mostly continuous and uniform layer lining the papillae throughout the benign lesion. Still, finding myoepithelial cells in some parts of a papillary lesion is not inconsistent with a diagnosis of carcinoma.[9–11] In IP, the adjacent ducts frequently show hyperplasia, whereas in EPC, the adjacent ducts are more likely to be involved by DCIS. The epithelial component in EPC is that of a uniform population of cells with hyperchromatic nuclei, lying

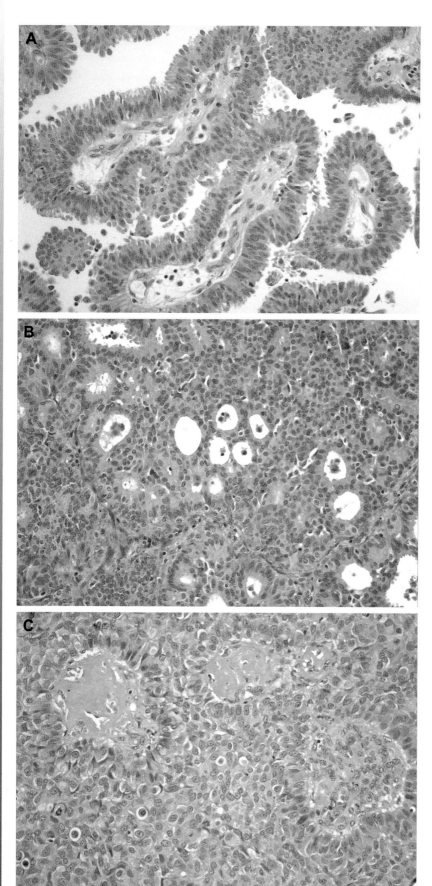

Fig. 6. Encapsulated papillary carcinoma (20 ×). The malignant epithelium lining the papillary scaffold grows as a single layer lining each core (A), proliferates between the cores to form cribriform structures (B), or grows as solid sheets of cells (C).

Fig. 7. Encapsulated papillary carcinoma (40 ×). The malignant epithelium consists of hyperchromatic nuclei, often low- to intermediate-grade with infrequent mitoses.

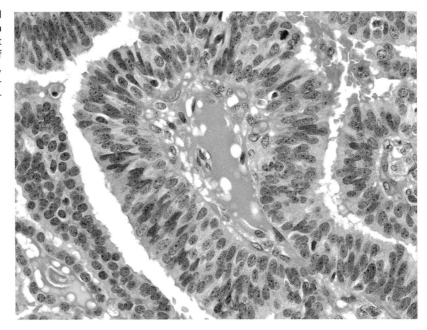

perpendicular to the fibrovascular stalks (**Fig. 17**A) or showing a solid, cribriform or micropapillary growth. This contrasts with the haphazard arrangement of cells with normochromatic nuclei, typical of IP (**Fig. 17**B).

Occasionally in EPC, an apparent second population of malignant epithelial cells can be present, which can mimic myoepithelial cells because of their frequently clear cytoplasm and their close proximity to the basement membrane (globoid cells). The presence of such a dimorphic population of cells in EPC, as described by Lefkowitz and colleagues,[4] can create diagnostic problems. The key to avoiding this error is in the

Fig. 8. Intraductal papilloma (2.5 ×). Low-power view showing a cystically dilated duct containing a papillary growth projecting into the duct lumen. Cytologic and architectural heterogeneity within the tumor is seen in contrast to the typical uniformity associated with encapsulated papillary carcinoma.

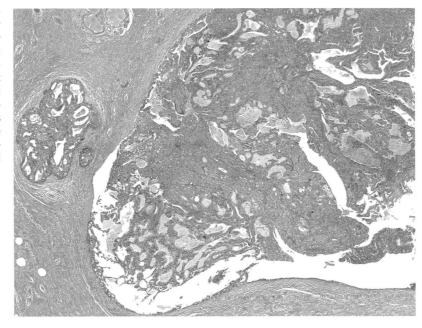

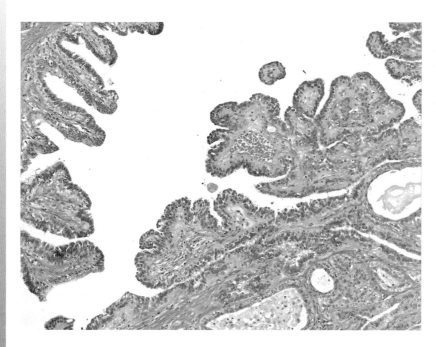

Fig. 9. Intraductal papilloma (10 ×). Branching fibrous cores containing central vessels form the basic structure on which myoepithelial and epithelial cells lie.

recognition of the cytologically atypical nuclei that resemble the adjacent malignant epithelial nuclei. Immunohistochemical stains can help confirm the epithelial rather than myoepithelial nature of these cells.

In sclerosing papillomas, there is increased collagenous stroma in the fibrovascular core and at the periphery of the lesion (**Fig. 18**). These lesions may appear more solid, and a definite cystic cavity may not be appreciated. Entrapped glandular elements may be found within the sclerosed cores and cystic duct wall that can mimic invasive carcinoma (**Fig. 19**). Although these glandular structures can be distorted, myoepithelial

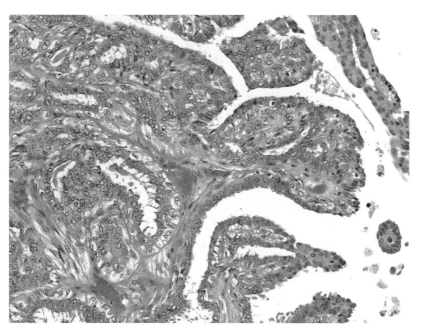

Fig. 10. Intraductal papilloma (20 ×). Each branch is lined by a layer of myoepithelial cells, which, as illustrated here, can have abundant clear cytoplasm. These are not always so conspicuous and may require immunohistochemical markers for their identification.

Fig.   11. Intraductal papilloma (20 ×). Lying on the layer of myoepithelium, at least one layer of benign epithelium is present. These are often cuboidal-to-columnar cells with a low nuclear-to-cytoplasmic ratio.

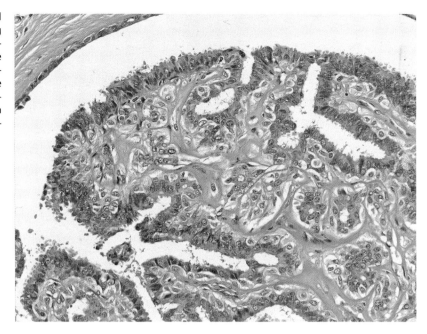

cells can be identified, and a hyalinized stroma typically surrounds the ducts rather than a desmoplastic stroma. That the underlying lesion is benign should prevent overdiagnosis of invasive carcinoma in this setting.

ATYPICAL DUCTAL HYPERPLASIA AND DUCTAL CARCINOMA IN SITU ARISING IN A BENIGN INTRADUCTAL PAPILLOMA

The epithelial component of an otherwise benign papilloma can be subject to a spectrum of

Fig. 12. Intraductal papilloma (5 × and 20 ×). The epithelium may proliferate between the fibrovascular cores to a variable extent. Here, florid epithelial hyperplasia of usual type is seen (*A*). Higher power

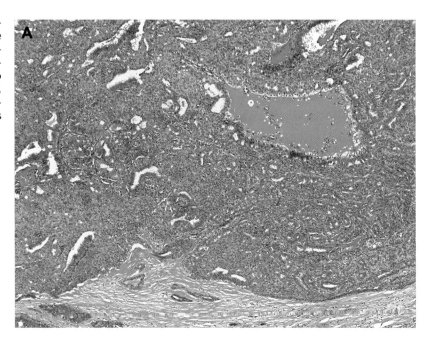

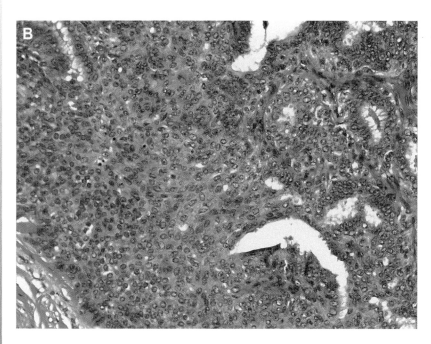

Fig. 12. (*B*) shows the typical morphology with overlapping nuclei, indistinct cell membranes, and streaming.

changes including metaplasia and hyperplasia, as described previously, but also ADH and in situ carcinoma. Typically these latter lesions have features of a benign intraductal papilloma with a focus or foci consisting of a neoplastic population of epithelial cells warranting the diagnosis of ADH or low-grade DCIS. These neoplastic foci are recognized as a uniform population of epithelial cells with round, hyperchromatic nuclei forming a rigid architecture with an absence of cellular streaming or overlapping (**Fig. 20**). Distinguishing such atypical areas from foci showing epithelial

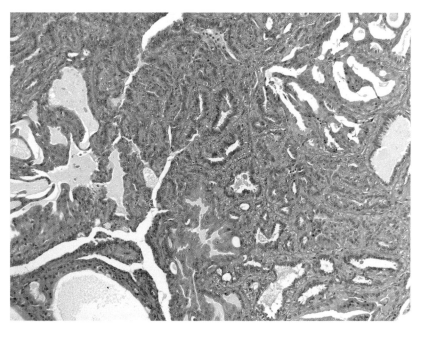

Fig. 13. Intraductal papilloma (10 ×). Apocrine metaplasia is frequently present. Large cells with abundant granular pink cytoplasm containing small round nuclei with nucleoli are seen.

Fig. 14. Intraductal papilloma (20 ×). Myoepithelial cells line each core and are present around the periphery of the dilated duct (*A*). These are highlighted with immunohistochemical staining for myoepithelial cells (smooth muscle myosin heavy chain/p63) (*B*).

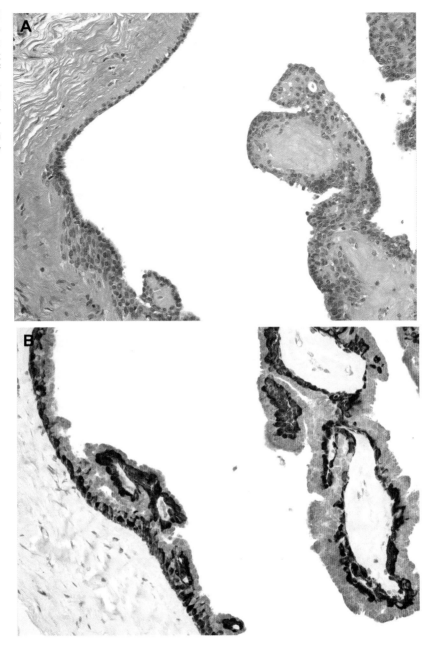

hyperplasia of usual type follows the criteria used in making this distinction outside the setting of a papilloma.[16,17]

Attempts at defining objective criteria that separate ADH from DCIS arising within a papilloma

have been made. Page and colleagues[18] have used size criteria with an arbitrary cut-off of 3 mm or less to distinguish ADH within a papilloma from DCIS within a papilloma. Tavassoli[19] has suggested the use of proportion criteria in evaluating

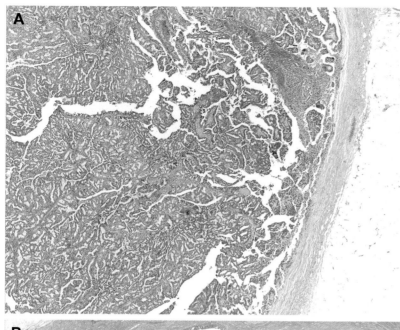

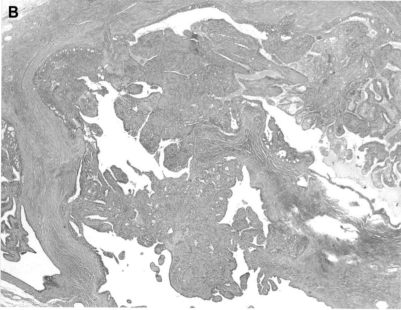

Fig. 15. Encapsulated papillary carcinoma versus intraductal papilloma (2.5 ×). Low-power view shows the delicate, less conspicuous cores that characterize the malignant lesion (*A*). In comparison, the cores that form the intraductal papilloma are fibrous and appear more pink on low power (*B*).

these lesions, with the term atypical papilloma applied when less than a third of the papilloma is involved by the atypical population and carcinoma in a papilloma if more than a third but less than 90% of the lesion shows such changes. Others have suggested that if the criteria for DCIS are met, whatever the extent, the lesion should be considered papilloma with DCIS.[20,21] These definitions are applied to low nuclear grade lesions only. The presence of higher-grade lesions is considered to represent carcinoma in a papilloma regardless of extent.

Fig. 16. Encapsulated papillary carcinoma (20 ×). While apocrine change is not a feature of encapsulated papillary carcinoma, apocrine differentiation can be seen. Cytologic atypia is identified and typically is similar to that seen in the nonapocrine appearing areas present in the rest of the tumor.

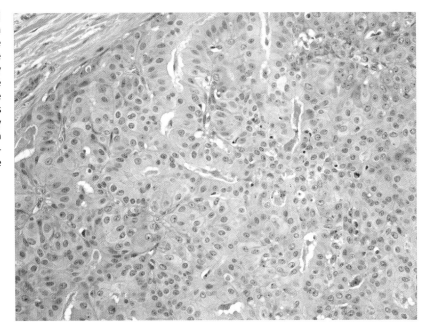

Little information is available regarding the clinical significance of the extent of atypia within a papilloma. In a study by MacGrogan and Tavassoli,[22] central papillomas were stratified according to the extent of atypia. There was found to be no significant difference in recurrence when the different categories were compared. The finding of usual hyperplasia, ADH, or lobular neoplasia in the surrounding breast parenchyma was, however, significantly associated with recurrences in the same breast. Overall, in patients treated with excision only, the number of events was small, which the authors suggest is a result of complete excision of the atypical cell population when confined to a localized lesion.

Page and colleagues[18] found a significant increase in risk (7.5-fold) of developing breast cancer in women who had ADH within a papilloma, and this risk was increased by the finding of ADH in the surrounding breast parenchyma. All but one of the invasive carcinomas arose in the ipsilateral breast; however, the numbers in this study were small. In contrast, subsequent studies[23,24] have found that the breast cancer risk associated with papillomas with atypia did not show an ipsilateral tendency, favoring that these lesions represent a generalized risk factor rather than a precursor lesion to breast cancer development. The risk in the larger of these studies was found to be five- and sevenfold for solitary and multiple papillomas, respectively.[23]

In summary, there is no consensus on the criteria for distinguishing ADH from DCIS arising in a papilloma. Furthermore, such a distinction is of questionable clinical importance. Complete excision with follow-up is appropriate, and decisions on further management of these patients should be made following assessment of the tissue surrounding the papilloma for an atypical epithelial proliferation.

SOLID PAPILLARY CARCINOMA

Solid papillary carcinoma (SPC) is sufficiently specific in its morphologic appearance and not infrequent association with mucinous carcinoma, to be discussed separately from EPC. The first reported case of the solid variant of papillary carcinoma was described by Rosen and Oberman,[25] and later the term SPC was coined by Maluf and Koerner.[26] The tumor typically is composed of well-circumscribed nodules of epithelial cells filling large or dilated ducts. Often extracellular mucin pools are present amidst the cellular proliferation (**Fig. 21**). Fibrovascular cores, frequently hyalinized, serve as the scaffold for the epithelial cells. Sclerosis of the stroma around and among the ducts is variably present, which can produce a pattern with features of a radial sclerosing lesion.[27] The cells are small to medium in size, ovoid-to-spindle-shaped and contain eosinophilic

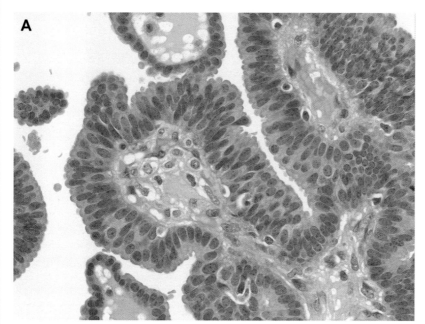

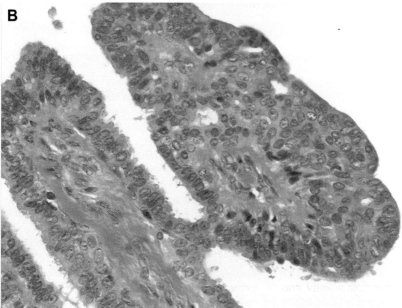

Fig. 17. Encapsulated papillary carcinoma versus intraductal papilloma (40 ×). A uniform population of epithelial cells with hyperchromatic nuclei lying perpendicular to the fibrovascular core is seen in encapsulated papillary carcinoma (A), in contrast to the haphazard arrangement of cells with normochromatic nuclei typical of intraductal papilloma (B).

cytoplasm. The nuclei contain fine chromatin with inconspicuous nucleoli. The cells polarize around the fibrovascular cores forming a palisade. Spindling is often marked with resultant streaming, and mitotic activity may be seen but is rarely greater than 10/10 high power fields (Fig. 22). Either intracellular or extracellular mucin is usually present and a signet-ring cell appearance can be seen. Associated invasive carcinoma is frequent, although often not the predominant lesion, and is mucinous carcinoma in 50% of cases.[28] In fact, based on the frequent association, Maluf and Koerner have proposed that SPC may be a precursor to mucinous carcinoma, cellular

Fig. 18. Sclerosing papilloma (2.5 ×). Increased collagenous stroma around the periphery of the papilloma rendering a more solid and distorted appearance.

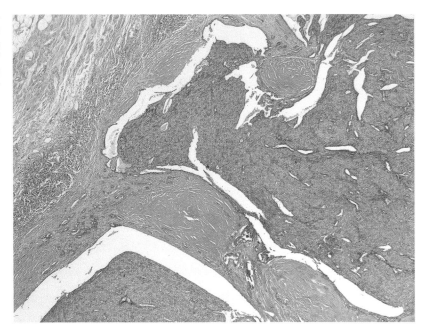

variant.[26] SPCs may be associated with other types of invasive carcinoma, including tumors showing neuroendocrine differentiation. In contrast, invasion associated with EPC is typically of ductal, no special type (NST).

The low-grade nuclei and streaming growth pattern can lead to a benign misdiagnosis. Morphologically, SPC can resemble UDH occurring within a papilloma. Both lesions share a papillary scaffold on which epithelial cells proliferate with a solid (or fenestrated) and streaming growth. Nuclear features shared by these lesions include cells with irregular nuclei, granular chromatin, and small nucleoli. SPC can be distinguished papilloma with UDH by the presence of a uniform population of cells with nuclear palisading around fibrovascular cores, increased mitotic activity, and the presence of intra- and extracellular mucin in the former.[26] Absence of CK5/6 staining in malignant proliferations and presence of staining in UDH have been shown to be of help in distinguishing these lesions.[29]

Whether SPC represents a mass-forming in situ lesion or an unconventional invasive carcinoma with a pushing border is unknown. In fact, immunohistochemistry for myoepithelial cells is typically negative around the periphery of the tumors, raising the possibility that these are truly invasive tumors.[26,30] In support of this is that metastases can be morphologically identical to the SPC component of the primary tumor.[26,28] These tumors, even when associated with unequivocal stromal invasion, tend to follow an indolent course.[26] A study by Nassar and colleagues[28] looked at outcome in 60 patients who had SPC with a mean follow-up of 9.4 years. When isolated, SPC was found to behave in an indolent manner, without lymph node or distant metastases. In patients who had SPC associated with invasion, 17.8% died of disease.

PAPILLARY DUCTAL CARCINOMA IN SITU

Papillary DCIS typically involves small- and medium-sized ducts and is usually more diffuse in its growth in contrast to the solitary EPC. The morphology is similar to what one sees in other forms of DCIS, but the architectural pattern is that of intraductal fibrovascular cores lined by malignant epithelium, showing varying degrees of proliferation (**Fig. 23**). Although absent from the intraductal proliferation, myoepithelial cells are present around the periphery of the duct, confirming their in situ nature. These lesions are managed as for other types of DCIS.

METASTATIC PAPILLARY CARCINOMA

Excluding the rare metastatic papillary thyroid or ovarian carcinoma is based on clinical history, the presence of an in situ component, and with the use of immunohistochemistry.

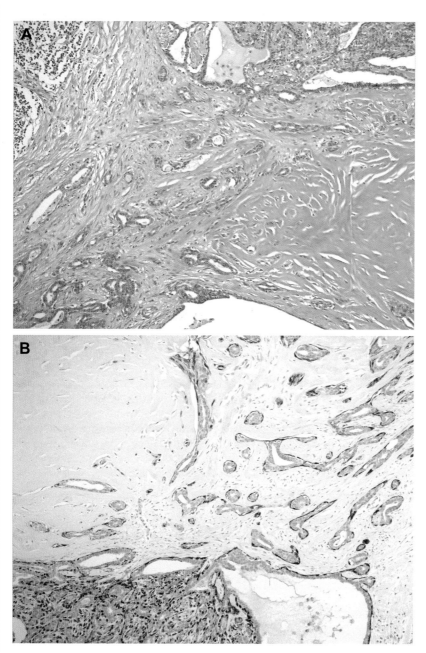

Fig. 19. Sclerosing papilloma (10 ×). The collagenous stroma can distort the periphery of the papilloma and entrap benign glands (*A*). Myoepithelial cells are preserved around the entrapped epithelium, and a desmoplastic stroma is not appreciated. Immunohistochemistry confirms the preservation of myoepithelial cells around the distorted glands (smooth muscle myosin heavy chain/p63) (*B*).

CARCINOMA WITH CYSTIC DEGENERATION

Carcinoma with cystic degeneration is a rare but important differential. Prognosis in such lesions differs from EPC, often being poor. High tumor grade, necrosis, and lack of true papillae in the former should facilitate in making the distinction.

INVASIVE PAPILLARY CARCINOMA

Fisher and colleagues[31] first used the term invasive papillary mammary cancer to describe a group of tumors that could be separated clearly from noninvasive papillary carcinoma. Prior to this, the term papillary carcinoma was used unqualified as

Fig. 20. Atypia within an intraductal papilloma (5 ×). The underlying lesion is that of a benign intraductal papilloma; however, focal architectural and cytologic atypia are present. The limited extent of the atypia (less than 3 mm) is in keeping with a diagnosis of atypical ductal hyperplasia within an intraductal papilloma. Of note, the atypical cells in this example contain eosinophilic cytoplasm, which stands out from the rest of the lesion.

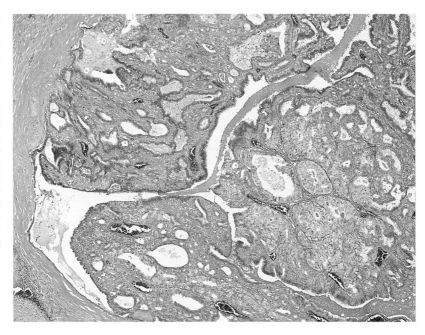

to its invasive or in situ nature. In their series, 35 of 1603 (2.1%) cancers from the National Surgical Adjuvant Breast Project were allocated to this category, making it a rare tumor.[31] These were found more commonly in older, non-Caucasian women.

Grossly, the appearances can vary, often being well-circumscribed and soft, although some may show sclerosis. Papillary formations within a desmoplastic stroma are the defining morphologic features (**Fig. 24**), and many can resemble papillary ovarian carcinoma or breast mucinous

Fig. 21. Solid papillary carcinoma (5 ×). Well-circumscribed nodules of tumor composed of sheets of malignant epithelial cells with fibrovascular cores are seen. Here, abundant extracellular mucin is present.

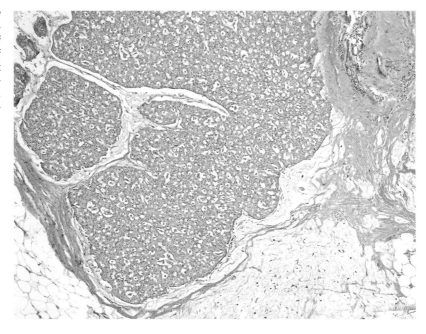

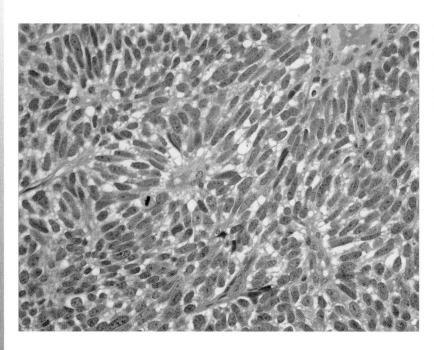

Fig. 22. Solid papillary carcinoma (40 ×). The cells are spindle-shaped and polarize around the fibrovascular cores. Mitotic figures are seen readily in this example.

carcinoma.[32] Mucin was present in approximately two-thirds of tumors in the original series.[31] Nuclei are typically grade 2 to 3. Cytoplasmic characteristics vary, but apocrine differentiation and apocrine snouts may be present.[32] Frequently, papillary or cribriform DCIS is seen adjacent to the tumor.

In the series of Fisher and colleagues,[31] 32% of patients had lymph node involvement. Overall, however, the 5-year disease free survival was approximately 90%. Only one of three patients who had recurrence died of disease, suggesting that this tumor behaves indolently.

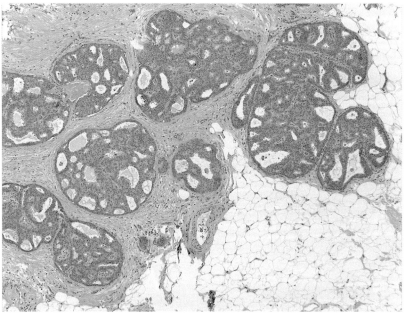

Fig. 23. Papillary ductal carcinoma in situ (5 ×). Numerous small- and medium-sized ducts are involved by an intraductal malignant proliferation characterized by the presence of fibrovascular cores. Myoepithelial cells are preserved around the periphery of the ducts. Other architectural forms of ductal carcinoma in situ often coexist.

Fig. 24. Invasive papillary carcinoma (2.5 ×). Variably sized papillary structures infiltrate through the stroma. Delicate fibrovascular cores and micropapillae are present.

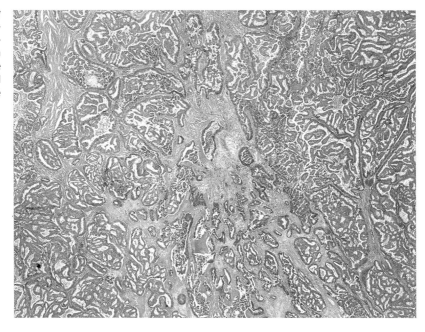

ENCAPSULATED PAPILLARY CARCINOMA WITH PSEUDO-INVASION AND INVASION

Many EPCs are bounded by zones of fibrosis, recent hemorrhage, and inflammation, probably secondary to injury as a result of torsion or prior tissue sampling (**Fig. 25**) that can lead to sclerosis with disruption of the regular, rounded contour.

Malignant epithelium can be found within such areas, and interpreting their significance is frequently problematic. A similar process of entrapment can be seen in benign counterparts. These pseudoinvasive nests typically run in parallel to the reactive stroma and capsule of the EPC. A desmoplastic response will be lacking. Immunohistochemical stains for myoepithelial

Fig. 25. Encapsulated papillary carcinoma (10 ×). Zones of fibrosis, hemorrhage, and inflammation surround the encapsulated papillary carcinoma. This is probably secondary to injury as a result of torsion or previous biopsy. This can lead to sclerosis with distortion of the regular contour.

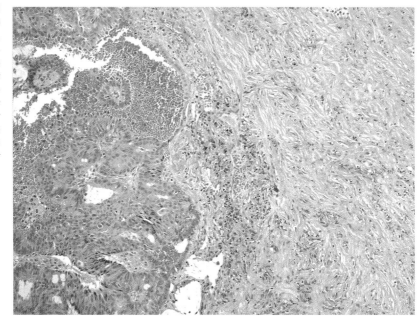

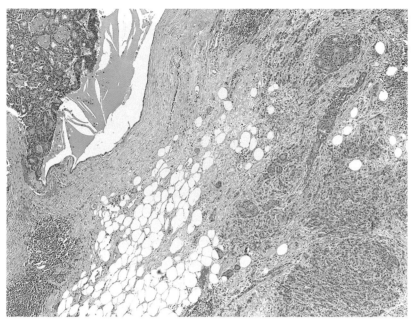

Fig. 26. Encapsulated papillary carcinoma with invasive ductal carcinoma, no special type (5 ×). When encapsulated papillary carcinoma (EPC) is associated with stromal invasion, it is typically invasive ductal, no special type. Here, residual EPC is seen in the upper left hand corner, and the invasive component is seen to extend into adjacent fat, beyond the zone of fibrosis. The invasive tumor stage is based on the largest focus of stromal invasion and does not include the encapsulated component.

cells are not usually helpful. The most reliable evidence for identifying invasion in these lesions is the presence of a recognizable pattern of invasive carcinoma extending beyond the zone of reactive stroma.

When stromal invasion can be recognized confidently, it is typically invasive ductal carcinoma, NST (**Fig. 26**) and not invasive papillary carcinoma. Measuring the extent of invasion is often difficult. The invasive focus alone should be used in determining the tumor stage. Not infrequently, however, multiple foci of stromal invasion are seen around the periphery of the tumor, and determining where the in situ component stops and invasion begins can be challenging. Including the entire lesion in the measurement is inappropriate, as such lesions would not be expected to behave as aggressively as tumors of equivalent size that are composed entirely of an invasive carcinoma. A common sense approach is needed, and each case should be dealt with on an individual basis.[33]

EPITHELIAL DISPLACEMENT

Papillary lesions that have been subjected to a previous needling procedure are prone to epithelial displacement.[34] This phenomenon involves displacement of epithelial fragments into the biopsy tract (**Fig. 27**A) or into lymphatic spaces (**Fig. 27**B), and they even can be transported mechanically to lymph nodes (benign mechanical transport).[35–37] Finding epithelial clusters within the site of the previous biopsy should prompt caution in making a diagnosis of invasive carcinoma, as in most instances, epithelial displacement will be the most likely diagnosis. Evidence of previous tissue manipulation is manifested by the presence of hemorrhage or hemosiderin, fibrosis, and inflammation. That papillary lesions are particularly prone to epithelial displacement, occurring in 94.3% cases in one study,[34] is likely a result of the inherent friability of the papillary cores.[34] Acknowledgment of such susceptibility should help prevent overdiagnosis of invasion in these instances. Features that help distinguish true lymph node metastasis from benign mechanical transport have been described. In the case of the latter, the epithelial clusters will be identical to the breast lesion and altered red blood cells and an inflammatory response, usually consisting of hemosiderin-laden macrophages, typically are seen.[35]

See **Table 1** for the histologic features used in differentiating between EPC and the entities in the differential diagnosis.

DIAGNOSIS

CLINICAL FEATURES

Encapsulated (intracystic) papillary carcinoma is rare, accounting for between 0.5% and 2% of all breast cancers[7,8,14,38] in women and representing a slightly greater percentage of overall breast

Fig. 27. Encapsulated papillary carcinoma and epithelial displacement. Following a needling procedure, epithelium can become displaced into the biopsy tract (*A*) (10 ×) or lymphatic channels (*B*) (20 ×), or it can be transported mechanically to axillary lymph nodes. Papillary lesions are particularly prone to this phenomenon, and recognizing this should avoid overdiagnosis of stromal invasion when epithelium is present within the biopsy site. The latter is evident by the presence of fibrosis, hemorrhage, or hemosiderin and inflammation.

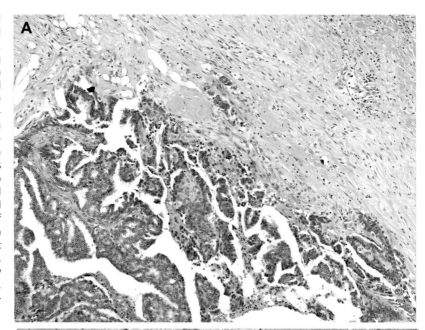

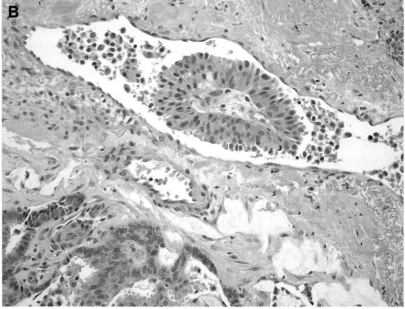

carcinoma in men.[27] Patients are typically older than those who have other types of carcinoma[4,39,40] and those who have benign IP. A mass lesion is present in up to 90% of patients.[19] Nearly half arise centrally in large ducts, and a nipple discharge, often blood-stained, occurs in at least one third of patients.[39,40] Most appear to grow slowly,[41] with symptoms reported for prolonged periods of time before diagnostic biopsy.[4,39,40,42]

RADIOLOGY

Mammographic findings with EPC are of a round or oval well-circumscribed mass with or without focal irregularity of the edges. Distinction from other well-circumscribed lesions such as a fibroadenoma, phyllodes tumor, and mucinous carcinoma can be difficult. Clustered microcalcifications are seen less frequently compared with papillary DCIS. On ultrasound, an indistinct border

Table 1
Differential diagnosis of encapsulated papillary carcinoma: histologic features used in differentiating between the entities

Feature	EPC	IP	ADH/DCIS in IP	SPC	Papillary DCIS	Invasive Papillary Carcinoma
Distribution	Often central, involving large ducts	Peripheral or central, multiple or solitary	As for IP	Often central, involving large ducts	Small- to medium-sized ducts, peripheral	–
Papillae	Delicate fibrovascular cores; less conspicuous than in IP	Fibrous cores, often abundant collagen	As for IP with focus/foci of atypia	Fibrovascular cores often inconspicuous due to solid proliferation of epithelium	Delicate fibrovascular cores	Delicate fibrovascular cores and micropapillae
Epithelial cytology and architecture	Uniform population of cells with hyperchromatic nuclei, often low-grade Varied architecture: single or multiple layers, cribriform, solid, micropapillary	Haphazard arrangement of benign epithelial cells with normochromatic nuclei, cuboidal to columnar in shape Varying degrees of epithelial hyperplasia of usual type	Atypical foci show low grade cytologic atypia; micropapillary, cribriform or solid architecture	Ovoid to spindle-shaped cells with inconspicuous nucleoli; fine chromatin, ± eosinophilic cytoplasm or signet-ring cells Solid sheets Streaming may be a feature	Malignant epithelial cells with variable nuclear grade; solid, cribriform or micropapillary patterns may be present	Usually low- to intermediate-grade cells Variable cytoplasm including apical snouts

Apocrine change	May show apocrine-like differentiation with eosinophilic cytoplasm but malignant nuclei	Common	Common in residual benign areas; atypical foci can show eosinophilic cytoplasm	–	–	Apocrine differentiation and apocrine snouts may be seen
Adjacent ducts	DCIS	Benign proliferations	Benign or atypical proliferations	DCIS	Frequently coexist with other patterns of DCIS	Papillary or cribriform DCIS frequent
Intraluminal myoepithelial cells	Absent	Present	Present in nonatypical areas; absent from within the atypical proliferation	Absent	Absent	Absent
Peripheral myoepithelial cells	Absent	Present	Present	Absent	Present	Absent
Associated invasive carcinoma	Typically ductal, NST	–	–	Frequently mucinous; also, ductal, NST ± neuroendocrine features	–	–

Abbreviations: ADH, atypical ductal hyperplasia; DCIS, ductal carcinoma in situ; EPC, encapsulated papillary carcinoma; IP, intraductal papilloma; SPC, solid papillary carcinoma; NST, no special type.

or microlobulation may be seen, which might suggest malignancy. EPCs often show a complex echo texture with both cystic and solid areas. The former may show septation with solid papillary masses projecting into the cystic lumen.[43] Radiologic appearances have been shown to be inaccurate in predicting benignancy or malignancy. Lam and colleagues[44] found sonography to be the more specific but slightly less sensitive modality than mammography. In this study, 8 of 21 (38%) lesions had discordance between imaging and histopathology.

When nipple discharge is the presenting symptom, galactography is a sensitive test to show intraductal filling defects, duct obstruction, and duct wall irregularity,[45] but it is not specific in terms of differentiating benign from malignant processes. Its rate of false positives and false negatives precludes its use as a reliable method to exclude malignancy and avoid surgery in benign cases.[46,47]

CORE BIOPSY

Papillary lesions account for between 0.73%[48] to 4%[49] of core biopsies. The nature of the lesion and the nature of the biopsy mean that the tissue available for evaluation frequently is fragmented, hampering interpretation. For example, florid epithelial hyperplasia of usual type represented out of context in a core biopsy can be misinterpreted as in situ carcinoma.[27] Particular challenges arise when residual benign IP coexists with a malignant component, the focal preservation of myoepithelial cells leading to confusion, and when evaluating malignant lesions for invasion. In the case of the latter, the presence of a monotonous population of epithelial cells lying directly on slender fibrovascular cores, without intervening myoepithelial cells, will clinch the diagnosis of malignancy, however, edge of the lesion may not be well-represented in the biopsy, and when it is, a reactive stroma with entrapped epithelium may be present (**Fig. 28**). Diagnosing invasive carcinoma in this setting warrants caution, and making a definitive diagnosis may need to be deferred until the lesion has been excised.

Although controversy remains as to whether all lesions diagnosed as benign IP on core biopsy need to be excised, there is general agreement that the presence of atypia within a papilloma should prompt excision because of the likelihood of finding DCIS in the resection specimen. Needless to say, biopsies with features to suggest EPC should prompt complete surgical excision.

IMMUNOHISTOCHEMISTRY IN DIAGNOSIS

Although evaluation of papillary lesions is based primarily on morphologic features, immunohistochemistry can be used as an adjunct to diagnosis. Interpretation of results must be done with caution, as several pitfalls can arise.

The presence of myoepithelial cells and their distribution in papillary lesions is particularly important. Several antibodies that decorate myoepithelial cells are available, including smooth muscle myosin heavy chain, smooth muscle actin, p63 and, calponin, each varying in sensitivity and specificity. Care must be taken in assessing their pattern of staining because of cross-reactivity with stromal myofibroblasts and pericytes surrounding blood vessels. Furthermore, some neoplastic cells in EPC can show positive staining with p63 and, when present at the periphery of the lesion, can be mistaken for myoepithelial cells.[2] Myoepithelial cells are preserved at the periphery of benign IP, IP with ADH/DCIS, and papillary DCIS; however, these are absent at the periphery of EPC (**Fig. 29**), SPC, and invasive papillary carcinoma and are not of value, therefore, in identifying true stromal invasion rather than pseudoinvasion in EPC or SPC.

Identifying a myoepithelial cell layer lining the fibrovascular cores is a key feature in distinguishing benign papillomas from EPC. In the former, each fibrovascular core is lined by a layer of myoepithelial cells on which the epithelial cells lie (**Fig. 30A**). The epithelium can proliferate to varying degrees in the space between the fibrovascular cores, but a myoepithelial cell layer separates this epithelial proliferation from the core. In contrast, in EPC, the epithelial component lies directly on the fibrovascular core without intervening myoepithelial cells (**Fig. 30B**). This is not always the case, however, and some EPCs can retain their intraluminal myoepithelial cells at least focally.[50–52] These most likely represent pre-existing benign intraductal papillomas that have become extensively involved by DCIS.[21] In such cases, the presence or absence of myoepithelial cells lining the fibrovascular cores cannot distinguish benign from malignant lesions reliably, and evaluation of the epithelial proliferation between the fibrovascular cores is key. Although this is based predominantly on morphologic features, several studies have evaluated the use of high molecular weight cytokeratins in this setting. In epithelial hyperplasia of usual type, the proliferation is of both luminal and basal cells, so staining for high molecular weight or basal cytokeratins (eg, CK 5 and CK 14) will be positive in most of the cells.

Fig. 28. Encapsulated papillary carcinoma, core biopsy (5 ×). Diagnosing the true nature of a papillary lesion on core biopsy can be challenging. Here, a uniform population of low-grade malignant epithelial cells lying on fibrovascular cores without intervening myoepithelial cells is seen. The adjacent stroma is reactive and should not be interpreted as representing the desmoplastic stroma seen with invasive carcinoma.

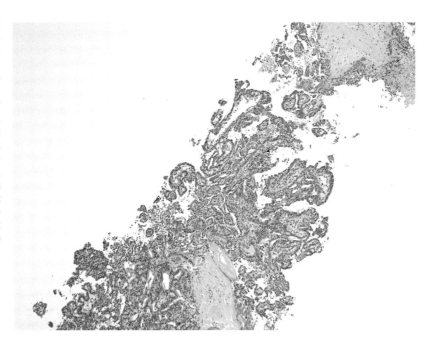

With low-grade neoplastic proliferations, however, the proliferating cells will be solely luminal and so, basal cytokeratin staining will be absent.[53–55] When applied to papillary lesions, a mosaic pattern of staining with high molecular weight cytokeratins is seen in IP with epithelial hyperplasia of usual type (**Fig. 31**A), whereas the foci of atypia in atypical papillomas show absence of staining (**Fig. 31**B).[56,57] Among the array of high molecular weight cytokeratins for use in distinguishing EPC from IP, CK5/6 has been shown to have the greatest sensitivity

Fig. 29. Encapsulated papillary carcinoma (smooth muscle myosin heavy chain) (20 ×). Myoepithelial cells are absent from the periphery of the tumor with immunohistochemical staining. Note the internal positive control with staining of myoepithelial cells around adjacent benign ducts.

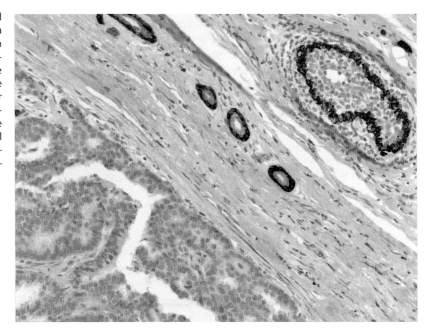

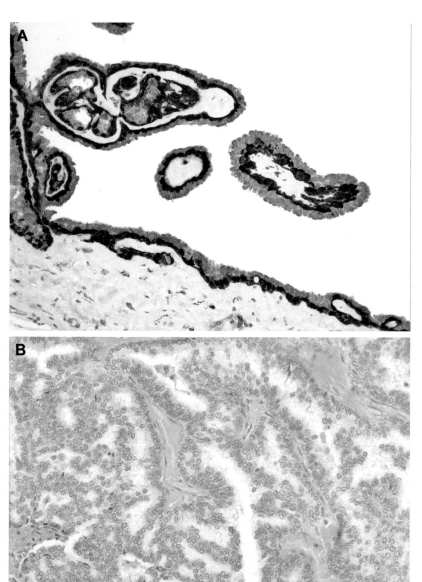

Fig. 30. Intraductal papilloma versus encapsulated papillary carcinoma (smooth muscle myosin heavy chain) (20 ×). The fibrovascular cores within the papillary network show preservation of myoepithelial cells along the papillae within intraductal papilloma (*A*). In contrast, fibrovascular cores show an absence of myoepithelial cells in encapsulated papillary carcinoma (*B*).

and negative predictive value and CK14 the greatest specificity and positive predictive value.[57]

Low-grade neoplastic proliferations typically show diffuse and uniform staining of the neoplastic population with estrogen receptor (**Fig. 31**C), in contrast to the variable pattern of staining seen in epithelial hyperplasia of usual type (**Fig. 31**D). Combining the results of ER staining with high molecular weight cytokeratin staining is useful in distinguishing ADH/low-grade DCIS from epithelial hyperplasia of usual type.[33]

Fig.   31. Intraductal papilloma with florid epithelial hyperplasia versus intraductal papilloma with atypia/ductal carcinoma in situ (10 ×). In areas of epithelial hyperplasia of usual type, a mosaic pattern of staining with high molecular weight cytokeratin is seen (CK5) (*A*). In an area of atypia, staining with high molecular weight cytokeratin is absent or minimal (CK5) (note internal positive control in the right of the image) (*B*).

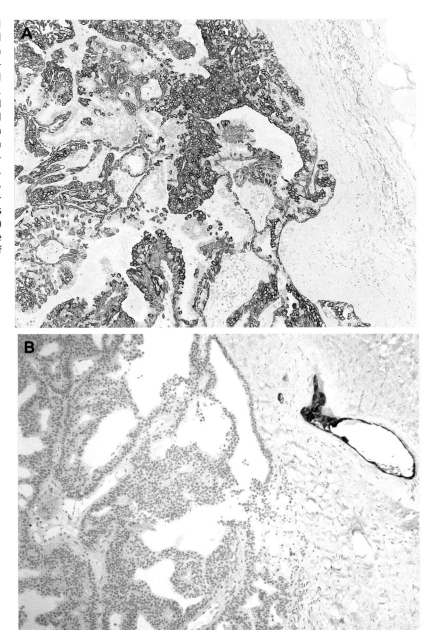

● Some reports suggest that DCIS can exhibit a basal-like phenotype.[58–60] Such cases are typically high-grade. In the rare occasions that this occurs within a papillary lesion, diffuse staining with high molecular weight cytokeratins will be seen. Complete absence of ER staining, however, will accompany this rather than the patchy ER staining seen with UDH (personal observation).

PROGNOSIS

Before Carter and colleagues[13] published their series of EPCs in 1983, several authors had looked at outcome in these patients but had failed to distinguish between invasive and noninvasive forms or those occurring with DCIS. For this reason, many concluded that the prognosis of these lesions was not good, and modified

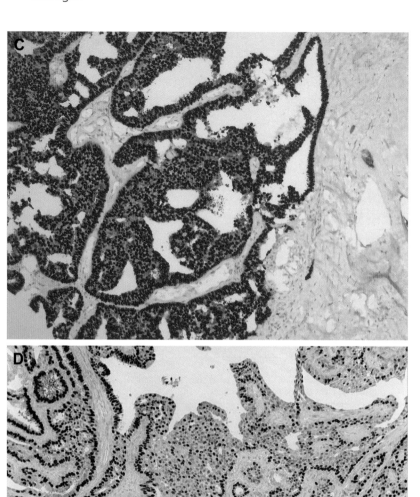

Fig. *31.* Estrogen receptor (ER). Diffuse strong staining with ER is seen in the area of atypia (*C*). In contrast, in the intraductal papilloma (same area as *A*), there is variable staining with ER (*D*).

radical mastectomy was considered the treatment of choice. Carter and colleagues' study suggested this was not the case. The authors separated papillary lesions into three groups: pure EPC, EPC with associated DCIS, and invasive papillary carcinoma. This study found that pure EPC, distinguished from EPC with either DCIS or invasion, had far less serious implications. Metastases or invasive recurrence did not feature with pure EPC at 14 years of follow-up. When associated with DCIS, EPC was more likely to be associated with recurrence and invasive recurrence. The number of patients in the study was small, however, with just 41 patients in total, 11 of whom had excision alone. Further evidence for the excellent outcome in patients who had pure EPC came from Harris and colleagues,[5] who reviewed 23 patients with a diagnosis of EPC. Only 1 of 14 patients with pure EPC had recurrence. This was in the form of pure EPC.

Metastases have been reported to rarely occur in patients who have EPC. Lefkowitz and colleagues[4] studied 77 such patients with 11.3 years mean follow-up. One patient with EPC without stromal invasion had axillary lymph node involvement at the time of surgery, and two other patients subsequently developed visceral metastases. Associated DCIS was found in two of three of these patients. Necrosis was present in one of the cases. Two were nuclear grade 2 and one nuclear grade 3. The Kaplan-Meier 5- and 10-year survival rates were 100%, and disease free survival was 96% and 91% respectively. Noteworthy is that 72 % patients in this study had undergone mastectomy.

In a similar study by Solorzano and colleagues,[61] four patients with either pure EPC or EPC with DCIS had local or distant recurrences. The one patient with pure EPC who experienced a recurrence had undergone a segmental mastectomy and received radiation. Her recurrence was local and represented a pure EPC. Of the three patients with recurrence who had EPC plus DCIS, one recurrence was local and DCIS only; one patient had a 2cm recurrence of papillary carcinoma in her axilla, and a third patient had bone metastases 7 years after local treatment. The disease-specific survival rate in this study was 100%, and the recurrence-free survival rate was 96%, 85%, and 77% at 2, 5, and 10 years, respectively. Disease-free survival did not differ significantly according to whether there was associated DCIS, invasive carcinoma, or pure EPC only. Nor did the extent of surgery or the administration of radiation therapy affect outcome.

One possible explanation for the rare occurrence of metastases in EPC, with or without DCIS, may be the presence of occult stromal invasion, missed as a result of inadequate sampling. A limitation of the study from Lefkowitz and colleagues[4] is that the tumors with metastases measured 3 cm, 2.5 cm, and 5cm, yet just four, three, and three sections were sampled from each of these lesions; hence, adequate exclusion of stromal invasion cannot be confirmed. Similarly, in the study by Solorzano and colleagues,[61] extent of sampling was not described. Recently, however, micrometastases to axillary lymph nodes have been reported in two cases of EPC, measuring 4 cm and 5.0 cm respectively, which either were sampled

extensively or completely embedded. Despite cutting multiple levels on several of the blocks, evidence of stromal invasion was not identified.[62] The lack of a basal myoepithelial cell layer suggests that these tumors might represent invasive cancers and might explain these exceedingly rare reports of metastases. Nonetheless, recurrences or metastases occurring in the setting of EPC without stromal invasion are rare, and the prognosis is excellent.

There remains a lack of consensus as to the optimal treatment of patients with EPC. Management trends have varied over time, with mastectomy, axillary lymph node dissection, and radiotherapy performed in many patients in earlier studies. More recent surgical approaches favor breast-conserving surgery (BCS). The low frequency of axillary lymph node metastases with pure EPC is felt to obviate the need for axillary lymph node dissection, but sentinel lymph node biopsy may be an alternative option for those patients who have large EPC.[62] In patients who have associated DCIS or invasion, adjuvant treatment should be based on the associated pathology; however, there is little consensus as to the roles that local radiation therapy or systemic endocrine therapy play in the treatment of isolated EPC. Fayanju and colleagues[63] looked at treatment in cases of EPC, either pure or with associated DCIS or invasion, and they found that patients with pure EPC in particular had very good outcomes even if the only therapy was surgery. Most mastectomies in their study were performed as a result of positive margins. All of these cases were EPC associated with DCIS. No patient with pure EPC had failed BCS.

Pitfalls
ENCAPSULATED PAPILLARY CARCINOMA

! A dimorphic population of cells may suggest the preservation of a myoepithelial cell layer lining the cores (globoid cells).

! Reactive stoma may mimic desmoplasia and stromal invasion.

! Neoplastic epithelium may become entrapped in fibrous capsule, mimicking stromal invasion.

! Prone to epithelial displacement following needling procedure—may lead to subsequent erroneous diagnosis of invasion/lymphatic invasion/lymph node metastases.

SUMMARY

Papillary carcinomas are rare, difficult to diagnose, classified in various ways and of uncertain prognosis. The true nature of EPCs has yet to be elucidated; however, the available evidence suggests that their behavior is likely to be indolent. Hence, classifying and staging these lesions as frankly invasive carcinomas should be avoided. Treatment should be conservative with complete surgical excision. Although those who have pure EPC may be candidates for adjuvant radiation therapy or endocrine therapy, the benefit of such treatments in this setting needs to be confirmed with prospective trials.

REFERENCES

1. Hill CB, Yeh IT. Myoepithelial cell staining patterns of papillary breast lesions: from intraductal papillomas to invasive papillary carcinomas. Am J Clin Pathol 2005;123(1):36–44.

2. Collins LC, Carlo VP, Hwang H, et al. Intracystic papillary carcinomas of the breast: a re-evaluation using a panel of myoepithelial cell markers. Am J Surg Pathol 2006;30(8):1002–7.

3. Leal C, Costa I, Fonseca D, et al. Intracystic (encysted) papillary carcinoma of the breast: a clinical, pathological, and immunohistochemical study. Hum Pathol 1998;29(10):1097–104.

4. Lefkowitz M, Lefkowitz W, Wargotz ES. Intraductal (intracystic) papillary carcinoma of the breast and its variants: a clinicopathological study of 77 cases. Hum Pathol 1994;25(8):802–9.

5. Harris KP, Faliakou EC, Exon DJ, et al. Treatment and outcome of intracystic papillary carcinoma of the breast. Br J Surg 1999;86(10):1274.

6. Czernobilsky B. Intracystic carcinoma of the female breast. Surg Gynecol Obstet 1967;124(1):93–8.

7. Gatchell FG, Dockerty MB, Clagett OT. Intracystic carcinoma of the breast. Surg Gynecol Obstet 1958;106(3):347–52.

8. McKittrick JE, Doane WA, Failing RM. Intracystic papillary carcinoma of the breast. Am Surg 1969; 35(3):195–202.

9. Murad TM, Swaid S, Pritchett P. Malignant and benign papillary lesions of the breast. Hum Pathol 1977;8(4):379–90.

10. Papotti M, Eusebi V, Gugliotta P, et al. Immunohistochemical analysis of benign and malignant papillary lesions of the breast. Am J Surg Pathol 1983;7(5):451–61.

11. Papotti M, Gugliotta P, Ghiringhello B, et al. Association of breast carcinoma and multiple intraductal papillomas: an histological and immunohistochemical investigation. Histopathology 1984;8(6):963–75.

12. Jaffer S, Chen X, Lee L, et al. Pleomorphic solid and cystic papillary carcinoma of the breast: two cases occurring in young women. Ann Diagn Pathol 2004;8(3):126–9.

13. Carter D, Orr SL, Merino MJ. Intracystic papillary carcinoma of the breast. After mastectomy, radiotherapy, or excisional biopsy alone. Cancer 1983; 52(1):14–9.

14. Kraus FT, Neubecker RD. The differential diagnosis of papillary tumors of the breast. Cancer 1962;15:444–55.

15. McDivitt RW, Stewart F, Berg JW. Tumors of the breast. In: Atlas of tumor pathology, 2nd series. Washington DC: Armed Forces of Pathology; 1968. p. 1–22.

16. Page DL, Rogers LW. Combined histologic and cytologic criteria for the diagnosis of mammary atypical ductal hyperplasia. Hum Pathol 1992;23(10):1095–7.

17. Tavassoli FA, Norris HJ. A comparison of the results of long-term follow-up for atypical intraductal hyperplasia and intraductal hyperplasia of the breast. Cancer 1990;65(3):518–29.

18. Page DL, Salhany KE, Jensen RA, et al. Subsequent breast carcinoma risk after biopsy with atypia in a breast papilloma. Cancer 1996;78(2):258–66.

19. Tavassoli FA. Papillary lesions. In: Pathology of the breast. 2nd edition. Stamford (CT): Appleton and Lange; 1999. p. 325–72.

20. Ellis IO, Elston CW, Pinder SE. Papillary lesions. In: Elston CW, Ellis IO, editors. The breast. Edinburgh (Scotland): Churchill Livingstone; 1998. p. 133–46.

21. Collins LC, Schnitt SJ. Papillary lesions of the breast: selected diagnostic and management issues. Histopathology 2008;52(1):20–9.

22. MacGrogan G, Tavassoli FA. Central atypical papillomas of the breast: a clinicopathological study of 119 cases. Virchows Arch 2003;443(5):609–17.

23. Lewis JT, Hartmann LC, Vierkant RA, et al. An analysis of breast cancer risk in women with single, multiple, and atypical papilloma. Am J Surg Pathol 2006;30(6):665–72.

24. Raju U, Vertes D. Breast papillomas with atypical ductal hyperplasia: a clinicopathologic study. Hum Pathol 1996;27(11):1231–8.

25. Rosen PP, Oberman HA. Tumors of the mammary gland. In: Atlas of tumor pathology, 3rd series. Washington DC: Armed Forces Institute of Pathology; 1993. p. 209–19.

26. Maluf HM, Koerner FC. Solid papillary carcinoma of the breast. A form of intraductal carcinoma with endocrine differentiation frequently associated with mucinous carcinoma. Am J Surg Pathol 1995; 19(11):1237–44.

27. Rosen PP. Papillary Carcinoma. In: Rosen's breast pathology. 2nd edition. Philadelphia: Lippincott Williams & Wilkins; 2001. p. 381–404.

28. Nassar H, Qureshi H, Volkanadsay N, et al. Clinico-pathologic analysis of solid papillary carcinoma of the breast and associated invasive carcinomas. Am J Surg Pathol 2006;30(4):501–7.

29. Rabban JT, Koerner FC, Lerwill MF. Solid papillary ductal carcinoma in situ versus usual ductal hyperplasia in the breast: a potentially difficult distinction resolved by cytokeratin 5/6. Hum Pathol 2006; 37(7):787–93.

30. Dickersin GR, Maluf HM, Koerner FC. Solid papillary carcinoma of breast: an ultrastructural study. Ultrastruct Pathol 1997;21(2):153–61.

31. Fisher ER, Palekar AS, Redmond C, et al. Pathologic findings from the National Surgical Adjuvant Breast Project (protocol no. 4). VI. Invasive papillary cancer. Am J Clin Pathol 1980;73(3):313–22.

32. Page DL, Anderson TJ. Uncommon types of invasive carcinoma. In: Diagnostic histopathology of the breast. London: Churchill Livingstone; 1987. p. 236–51.

33. Mulligan AM, O'Malley FP. Papillary lesions of the breast: a review. Adv Anat Pathol 2007;14(2): 108–19.

34. Nagi C, Bleiweiss I, Jaffer S. Epithelial displacement in breast lesions: a papillary phenomenon. Arch Pathol Lab Med 2005;129(11):1465–9.

35. Carter BA, Jensen RA, Simpson JF, et al. Benign transport of breast epithelium into axillary lymph nodes after biopsy. Am J Clin Pathol 2000;113(2): 259–65.

36. Youngson BJ, Cranor M, Rosen PP. Epithelial displacement in surgical breast specimens following needling procedures. Am J Surg Pathol 1994;18(9): 896–903.

37. Youngson BJ, Liberman L, Rosen PP. Displacement of carcinomatous epithelium in surgical breast specimens following stereotaxic core biopsy. Am J Clin Pathol 1995;103(5):598–602.

38. Framarino dei Malatesta ML, Piccioni MG, Felici A, et al. Intracystic carcinoma of the breast. Our experience. Eur J Gynaecol Oncol 1992;13(Suppl 1): 40–4.

39. Carter D. Intraductal papillary tumors of the breast: a study of 78 cases. Cancer 1977;39(4):1689–92.

40. Haagensen CD. Papillary breast carcinoma. In: Diseases of the breast. 2nd edition. Philadelphia: WB Saunders; 1971. p. 528–44.

41. Meyer JS, Bauer WC, Rao BR. Subpopulations of breast carcinoma defined by S-phase fraction, morphology, and estrogen receptor content. Lab Invest 1978;39(3):225–35.

42. Hunter CE Jr, Sawyers JL. Intracystic papillary carcinoma of the breast. Southampt Med J 1980;73(11): 1484–6.

43. Knelson MH, el Yousef SJ, Goldberg RE, et al. Intracystic papillary carcinoma of the breast: mammographic, sonographic, and MR appearance with pathologic correlation. J Comput Assist Tomogr 1987;11(6):1074–6.

44. Lam WW, Chu WC, Tang AP, et al. Role of radiologic features in the management of papillary lesions of the breast. AJR Am J Roentgenol 2006;186(5): 1322–7.

45. Cardenosa G, Doudna C, Eklund GW. Ductography of the breast: technique and findings. AJR Am J Roentgenol 1994;162(5):1081–7.

46. King TA, Carter KM, Bolton JS, et al. A simple approach to nipple discharge. Am Surg 2000; 66(10):960–6.

47. Simmons R, Adamovich T, Brennan M, et al. Nonsurgical evaluation of pathologic nipple discharge. Ann Surg Oncol 2003;10(2):113–6.

48. Renshaw AA, Derhagopian RP, Tizol-Blanco DM, et al. Papillomas and atypical papillomas in breast core needle biopsy specimens: risk of carcinoma in subsequent excision. Am J Clin Pathol 2004; 122(2):217–21.

49. Rubin E, Dempsey PJ, Pile NS, et al. Needle-localization biopsy of the breast: impact of a selective core needle biopsy program on yield. Radiology 1995;195(3):627–31.

50. Putti TC, Pinder SE, Elston CW, et al. Breast pathology practice: most common problems in a consultation service. Histopathology 2005;47(5): 445–57.

51. Raju U, Crissman JD, Zarbo RJ, et al. Epitheliosis of the breast. An immunohistochemical characterization and comparison to malignant intraductal proliferations of the breast. Am J Surg Pathol 1990; 14(10):939–47.

52. Soini Y, Miettinen M. Immunohistochemical evaluation of the cytoarchitecture of benign and malignant breast lesions. APMIS 1992;100(10):901–7.

53. Nagle RB, Bocker W, Davis JR, et al. Characterization of breast carcinomas by two monoclonal antibodies distinguishing myoepithelial from luminal epithelial cells. J Histochem Cytochem 1986;34(7): 869–81.

54. Bocker W, Bier B, Freytag G, et al. An immunohistochemical study of the breast using antibodies to basal and luminal keratins, alpha-smooth muscle actin, vimentin, collagen IV and laminin. Part II: epitheliosis and ductal carcinoma in situ. Virchows Arch A Pathol Anat Histopathol 1992;421(4):323–30.

55. Gown AM, Vogel AM. Monoclonal antibodies to human intermediate filament proteins. II. Distribution of filament proteins in normal human tissues. Am J Pathol 1984;114(2):309–21.

56. Ichihara S, Fujimoto T, Hashimoto K, et al. Double immunostaining with p63 and high molecular weight cytokeratins distinguishes borderline papillary lesions of the breast. Pathol Int 2007;57(3):126–32.

57. Tan PH, Aw MY, Yip G, et al. Cytokeratins in papillary lesions of the breast: is there a role in distinguishing

intraductal papilloma from papillary ductal carcinoma in situ? Am J Surg Pathol 2005;29(5):625–32.

58. Bryan BB, Schnitt SJ, Collins LC. Ductal carcinoma in situ with basal-like phenotype: a possible precursor to invasive basal-like breast cancer. Mod Pathol 2006;19(5):617–21.

59. Dabbs DJ, Chivukula M, Carter G, et al. Basal phenotype of ductal carcinoma in situ: recognition and immunohistologic profile. Mod Pathol 2006; 19(11):1506–11.

60. Livasy CA, Perou CM, Karaca G, et al. Identification of a basal-like subtype of breast ductal carcinoma in situ. Hum Pathol 2007;38(2):197–204.

61. Solorzano CC, Middleton LP, Hunt KK, et al. Treatment and outcome of patients with intracystic papillary carcinoma of the breast. Am J Surg 2002; 184(4):364–8.

62. Mulligan AM, O'Malley FP. Metastatic potential of encapsulated (intracystic) papillary carcinoma of the breast: a report of 2 cases with axillary lymph node micrometastases. Int J Surg Pathol 2007; 15(2):143–7.

63. Fayanju OM, Ritter J, Gillanders WE, et al. Therapeutic management of intracystic papillary carcinoma of the breast: the roles of radiation and endocrine therapy. Am J Surg 2007;194(4):497–500.

USE OF MYOEPITHELIAL CELL MARKERS IN THE DIFFERENTIAL DIAGNOSIS OF BENIGN, IN SITU, AND INVASIVE LESIONS OF THE BREAST

Adriana D. Corben, MD[a,b], Melinda F. Lerwill, MD[a,b],*

KEYWORDS

- Breast • Myoepithelial cell • Invasive carcinoma • In situ carcinoma
- Smooth muscle actin • Calponin • Smooth muscle myosin heavy chain • p63

ABSTRACT

Immunohistochemical markers for myoepithelial cells are commonly used to distinguish invasive from noninvasive lesions in the breast. The approach takes advantage of the fact that conventional invasive carcinomas lack surrounding myoepithelial cells, whereas nearly all benign lesions and in situ carcinomas retain their myoepithelial cell layer. Although conceptually straightforward, the interpretation of myoepithelial cell markers can be complicated by misleading patterns of reactivity (such as stromal or tumor cell staining) or lack of reactivity (due to reduced numbers of myoepithelial cells or variable antigenicity). In this article, we discuss the advantages and disadvantages of commonly used myoepithelial cell markers, their general utility in distinguishing invasive from noninvasive processes, and pitfalls in their interpretation. We also examine whether the detection of myoepithelial cells is helpful in the evaluation of papillary lesions, another common application. Myoepithelial cell markers can be diagnostically useful in the distinction of many benign, in situ, and invasive lesions, but they must be interpreted in conjunction with careful morphologic analysis.

The glandular tree of the breast is invested by a peripheral layer of myoepithelial cells. The myoepithelial cells lie between the luminal epithelial cells and the basement membrane, forming a longitudinally oriented sheath along the ducts and a basket-like network around the acini.[1] Myoepithelial cells play a critical role in many diverse biologic events, including mammary morphogenesis, lactation, and neoplasia.[2] Although our understanding of their role in breast cancer is rudimentary, current evidence suggests that normal myoepithelial cells have a tumor suppressor–type function, and that alterations in the myoepithelial cell layer are associated with molecular alterations in the overlying glandular epithelium.[3–6] It is likely that a complex interplay between the myoepithelial cells, luminal cells, and stroma contributes to the microenvironment that governs both the establishment of intraductal malignancy and the progression to invasive carcinoma.

In order for a carcinoma to become invasive, the tumor cells must breach the myoepithelial cell layer and basement membrane surrounding a duct or acinus. Accordingly, the invasive tumor lacks surrounding myoepithelial cells (**Fig. 1**). From the pathologist's perspective, this observation can be exploited to address the sometimes difficult

[a] James Homer Wright Pathology Laboratories of the Massachusetts General Hospital, 55 Fruit Street, Boston, MA 02114, USA
[b] Department of Pathology, Harvard Medical School, 25 Shattuck Street, Boston, MA 02115, USA
* Corresponding author.
E-mail address: mlerwill@partners.org (M.F. Lerwill).

Surgical Pathology 2 (2009) 351–373
doi:10.1016/j.path.2009.02.003
1875-9181/09/$ – see front matter © 2009 Published by Elsevier Inc.

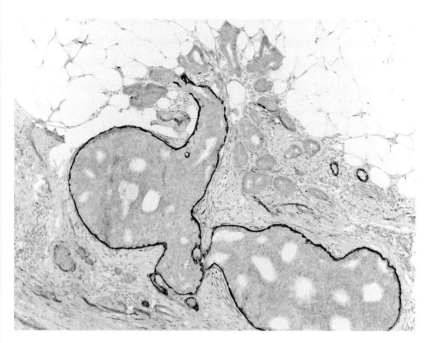

Fig. 1. Early invasive ductal carcinoma, focally still in continuity with the ductal carcinoma in situ from which it arose. The invasive component no longer has a surrounding layer of calponin-positive myoepithelial cells.*

diagnostic question of whether or not there is stromal invasion. The presence of an intact myoepithelial layer supports an intraductal process, whereas its absence indicates invasion. Myoepithelial cells can be recognized on routine hematoxylin- and eosin-stained sections, but they are not always easily identifiable. Furthermore, flattened tumor cells or stromal cells may mimic them in appearance, and confident confirmation of their absence is histologically difficult. Immunohistochemical stains for myoepithelial antigens are therefore commonly used to verify the presence or absence of the myoepithelial cell layer (**Fig. 2**). These markers are invaluable diagnostic tools, but their interpretation is frequently complicated by misleading or unexpected patterns of reactivity or nonreactivity. To avoid misdiagnosis, one must be aware of the many interpretive pitfalls associated with these immunohistochemical markers.

MYOEPITHELIAL CELL MARKERS

Myoepithelial cells contain smooth muscle–type cytoskeletal and contractile proteins that confer the contractile function necessary for milk ejection during lactation. Many of the antibodies used to detect myoepithelial cells are directed against these smooth muscle components, which are localized to the cytoplasm. Smooth muscle actin, calponin, and smooth muscle myosin heavy chain are three such markers that are widely employed. All are highly sensitive for the detection of

> ### *Key Features*
> #### MYOEPITHELIAL CELL MARKERS
>
> 1. Immunohistochemical stains to detect myoepithelial cells can be helpful for distinguishing benign and in situ lesions from invasive carcinoma.
>
> 2. Misinterpretation of stromal myofibroblast staining for evidence of a myoepithelial cell layer is a common error.
>
> 3. Each of the commonly used myoepithelial cell markers has its own advantages and disadvantages, thus a panel is suggested for complementary interpretation: at least one of the smooth muscle markers (preferably calponin or smooth muscle myosin heavy chain), p63, cytokeratin, and a matched hematoxylin- and eosin-stained section.
>
> 4. In the evaluation of intraductal papillary lesions, the cytologic features of the epithelial cells are more important than the number of myoepithelial cells.
>
> 5. When using myoepithelial cell markers, be aware of the potential interpretive pitfalls and always correlate the findings with morphology.

Fig. 2. (*A*) Invasive ductal carcinoma mimicking benign adenosis. (*B*) An immunostain for smooth muscle myosin heavy chain confirms an absence of myoepithelial cells. Blood vessels serve as an internal positive control.

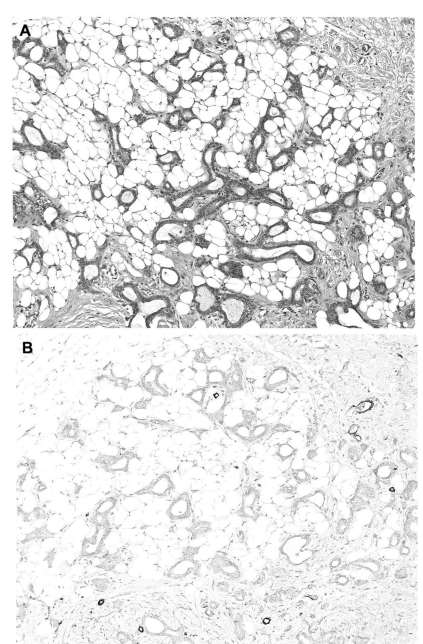

myoepithelial cells, although smooth muscle actin and calponin are slightly more sensitive than smooth muscle myosin heavy chain.[7] Notably, all three also crossreact with stromal myofibroblasts. Smooth muscle actin demonstrates the greatest amount of myofibroblast staining and smooth muscle myosin heavy chain the least.[7]

Periductal stromal staining can lead one to conclude that a myoepithelial cell layer is present when in fact it is not. Indeed, the degree of stromal staining with smooth muscle actin is such that we do not recommend its routine usage. The smooth muscle markers also stain blood vessels, and smooth muscle myosin heavy chain reacts with follicular dendritic cells in germinal centers. Benign and malignant epithelial cells are rarely immunoreactive for these markers.

p63, a homolog of p53, is an important developmental regulator and is expressed in the basal epithelia of many adult tissues, including the myoepithelial cells of the breast.[8] p63 is a sensitive marker for myoepithelial cells, demonstrating a nuclear staining pattern that gives a dotted-line effect (see **Fig. 12**A). Quite helpfully, p63 is not expressed in either stromal myofibroblasts or blood vessels, and therefore it usually yields a "cleaner" result than the smooth muscle markers. p63 is, however, occasionally positive in benign and malignant epithelial cells, especially high-grade ductal carcinomas.[7–11]

Mammary myoepithelial cells also express a variety of other antigens. CD10 reacts with myoepithelial cells[12] but, in our experience, is not as sensitive as the above-mentioned smooth muscle markers or p63. CD10 also stains stromal myofibroblasts. High molecular weight cytokeratins, such as cytokeratins 5 and 14, are expressed in myoepithelial cells and not in the stroma.[13] However, we have found these cytokeratins to be variably reactive in the normal myoepithelium,

with many immunonegative myoepithelial cells, and thus we do not consider them as reliable as other markers. High molecular weight cytokeratins are also frequently expressed in luminal cells, and epithelial positivity can make it more difficult to appreciate the presence or absence of myoepithelial cell staining. S-100 has been used for the detection of myoepithelial cells, but it is only a moderately sensitive marker and is frequently immunoreactive in both normal and neoplastic luminal cells.[14] Maspin, Wilms' tumor-1, P-cadherin, and D2-40 are also expressed in mammary myoepithelial cells.[15–17] They do not appear to be superior to the smooth muscle markers or p63 for routine diagnostic purposes, and the latter are generally more readily available in pathology laboratories. The following discussion focuses primarily on the smooth muscle markers and p63, as these are the most widely used.

PITFALLS IN INTERPRETATION

Immunohistochemical stains for myoepithelial markers are often straightforward to interpret: benign lesions and in situ carcinomas have a peripheral rim of positive cells, whereas invasive carcinomas are negative (see **Fig. 2**). Misleading or confusing staining patterns, however, are a regular occurrence. The reasons for interpretive difficulty range from the common (ie, stromal myofibroblast staining) to the exotic (ie, lack of myoepithelial cells as an intrinsic property of microglandular adenosis). Careful correlation of the morphologic and immunohistochemical findings is critical for correct diagnosis.

STAINING OF NONMYOEPITHELIAL CELLS

The propensity of stromal myofibroblasts to react with the smooth muscle–based markers can lead to a misdiagnosis of in situ carcinoma when the carcinoma is actually invasive. Invasive tumor nests may have closely apposed myofibroblasts, and when the latter stain positively, they can give the false impression of a surrounding myoepithelial cell layer (**Figs. 3** and **4**). This is the most common source of interpretive error in the evaluation of myoepithelial cell markers. Attention to morphologic features will help one to avoid this pitfall. Myofibroblasts have a purely linear staining pattern (**Fig. 5**A). Myoepithelial cells, on the other hand, bulge toward the luminal cells and interdigitate slightly (**Fig. 5**B). Their elongate cytoplasmic processes may appear linear, but their cell bodies form small bumps or triangular shapes that are identifiable along the course of the myoepithelial

Pitfalls

INTERPRETATION OF MYOEPITHELIAL CELL MARKERS

! Failure to recognize an invasive carcinoma can result from

   a. Periductal myofibroblast staining mimicking a myoepithelial cell layer

   b. Periductal blood vessel staining mimicking a myoepithelial cell layer

   c. Tumor cell staining mimicking a myoepithelial cell layer

   d. Failure to identify immunonegative invasive foci

! An overdiagnosis of stromal invasion can result from

   a. Myoepithelial cell layer attenuation

   b. Absence of myoepithelial cells in certain benign conditions

   c. Failure of myoepithelial cells to react with certain antibodies (variable antigenicity)

Fig. 3. Invasive carcinoma misdiagnosed as ductal carcinoma in situ. (*A*) Prominent myofibroblast staining around the invasive nests was misinterpreted as evidence of a myoepithelial cell layer on a smooth muscle actin immunostain. (*B*) A p63 immunostain on a deeper level confirms an absence of myoepithelial cells. A few benign ductules with intact myoepithelium are present.

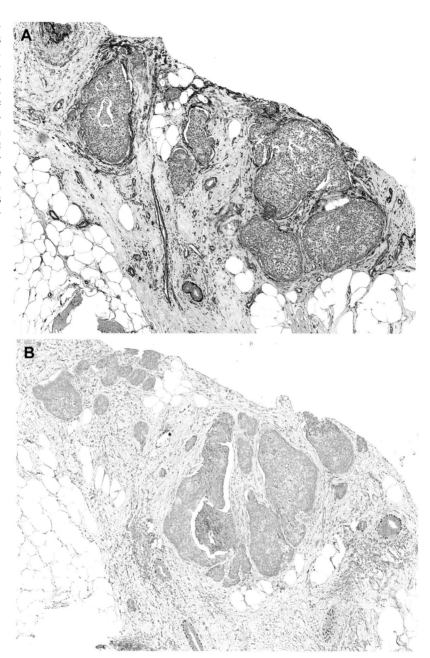

cell layer. The presence of a purely linear staining pattern should therefore raise concern that the immunoreactive cells are stromal in nature, especially if there is also adjacent stromal staining. Using a marker with less myofibroblast reactivity, such as smooth muscle myosin heavy chain, or one with no myofibroblast reactivity, such as p63, can be illuminating (see **Fig. 3**).

Blood vessels also stain for the smooth muscle-based markers. On occasion, this can lead to diagnostic difficulty because invasive tumor nests can be surrounded by a rim of small capillaries. The

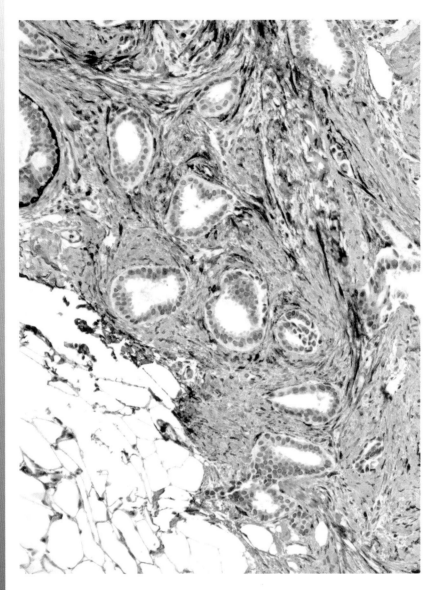

Fig. 4. Invasive tubular carcinoma with juxtaposed smooth muscle actin–positive myofibroblasts. The findings were misinterpreted as evidence of a partial myoepithelial cell layer.

lumina may be tiny and inconspicuous. As with my-ofibroblasts, staining of these vessels can lead to misinterpretation of an intact myoepithelial cell layer. This can be a pitfall in tumors with a rich vascular component, such as invasive papillary carcinomas. Attention to the morphology of the immunoreactive cells, correlation with the findings on routine stains, and usage of p63, which does not stain blood vessels, will help one to avoid misinterpretation.

Both benign and malignant epithelial cells can react with myoepithelial cell markers.

Immunoreactive benign and in situ carcinoma cells are generally not a source of interpretive difficulty, because they are still surrounded by a distinct myoepithelial cell layer. Immunoreactive invasive tumor cells, however, may be mistaken for benign myoepithelial cells and lead to misdiagnosis of an in situ process. p63 is more problematic than the smooth muscle markers in this regard; up to 12% of invasive carcinomas have p63-positive cells.[7–11] p63 reactivity is seen most frequently in poorly differentiated carcinomas and those with squamous differentiation, and only occasionally

Fig. 5. (*A*) Purely linear staining pattern due to stromal myofibroblasts. (*B*) True myoepithelial cells bulge toward and interdigitate slightly with the epithelial cells. (*A, B*: calponin immunostains).

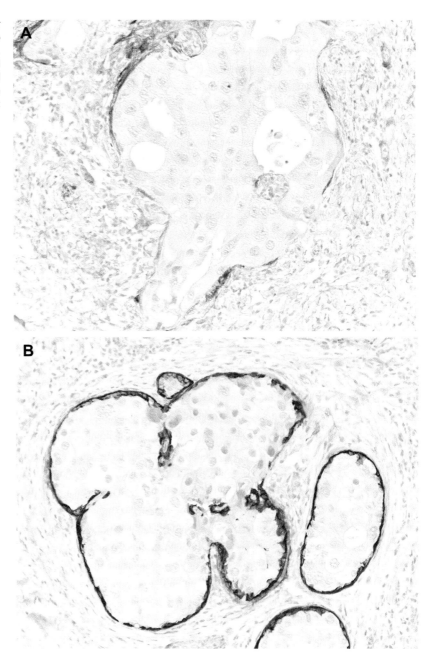

in low-grade carcinomas. The distribution and morphology of the positive tumor cells facilitate their distinction from myoepithelial cells. Immunoreactive tumor cells tend to be focal, not restricted to the periphery of the tumor nests, and larger than myoepithelial cells (**Fig. 6**). They have the same nuclear morphology as adjacent tumor cells. Curiously, low-grade papillary carcinomas sometimes demonstrate p63-positive tumor cells at the tumor periphery, near the expected location of myoepithelial cells.[11] The columnar morphology of the positive cells distinguishes them from myoepithelial cells.

Certain subtypes of invasive carcinoma in the breast demonstrate myoepithelial differentiation and thus will stain for myoepithelial markers.

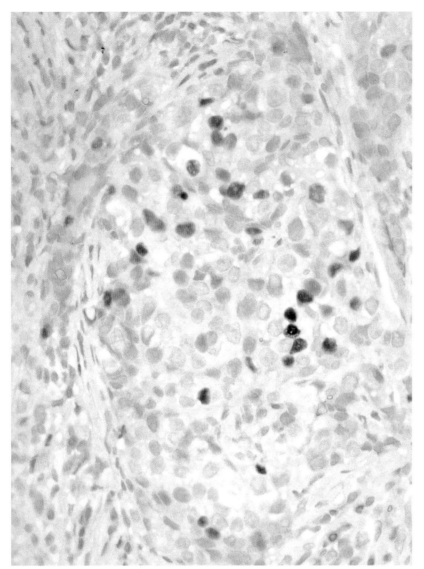

Fig. **6.** p63-positive tumor cells are not localized to the periphery of the tumor nest, and they demonstrate significant cytologic atypicality.

These include low-grade adenosquamous carcinoma, adenoid cystic carcinoma, malignant adenomyoepithelioma, and myoepithelial carcinoma. Of these, low-grade adenosquamous carcinoma is the most likely to be evaluated with myoepithelial markers to confirm invasion, and the most likely to give confusing results. In this tumor, the malignant myoepithelial cells are often located at the periphery of the invasive nests, simulating the location of benign myoepithelial cells (**Fig. 7**). Additionally, the squamous cells express p63. Thus there may be a significant amount of immunoreactivity in the tumor, in a pattern that may superficially mimic an intact myoepithelial cell layer (**Fig. 8A**). Several unusual staining patterns are typically encountered, however, that should raise concern that the positive cells are neoplastic. First, the presence of several layers of immunoreactive cells within individual tumor nests (**Fig. 8A**) suggests a neoplastic process rather than normal myoepithelium, which is composed of a single cell layer. Second, variable reactivity for different markers often occurs in neoplastic myoepithelial cells. For example,

Fig. 7. Low-grade adenosquamous carcinoma. A smooth muscle myosin heavy chain immunostain highlights peripheral myoepithelial differentiation in the invasive tumor nests.

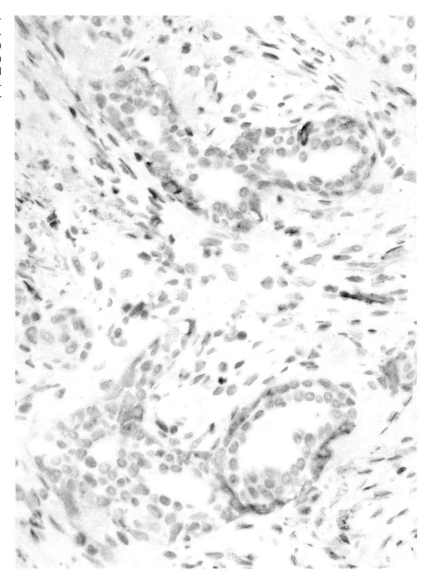

some tumor cells may be positive for multiple markers, such as calponin, smooth muscle myosin, and p63, whereas other cells in the same tumor may react with only one of the markers. Also, the squamous cells in low-grade adenosquamous carcinoma stain for p63 but not for the smooth muscle markers (**Fig.** 8A, B). Third, tumor nests that are completely negative for myoepithelial cells are usually readily found. These aberrant patterns of reactivity can provide a helpful hint to the neoplastic nature

of the immunoreactive cells. Ultimately, though, the diagnosis rests on careful morphologic evaluation, and in this context, myoepithelial markers are of limited utility for the assessment of invasion.

OVERLOOKED FOCI OF INVASION

The second most common source of diagnostic error arises not from the misinterpretation of positively staining cells, but rather from the failure to

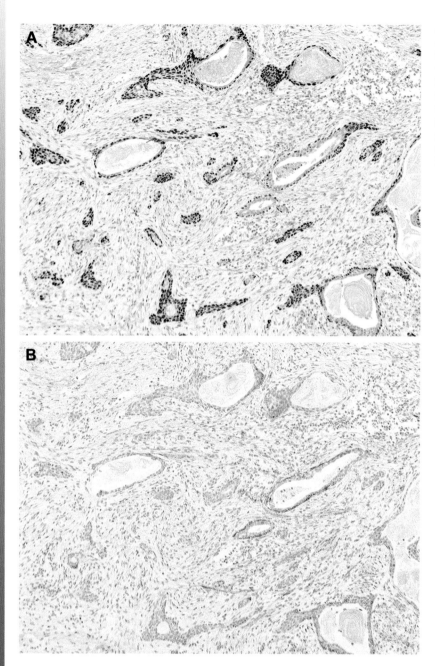

Fig. 8. Low-grade adenosquamous carcinoma. (*A*) Extensive reactivity for p63 with multilayering of the positive tumor cells. Some but not all of the labeled cells are squamous. (*B*) Smooth muscle myosin heavy chain is mostly negative in the same area.

identify invasive foci that are appropriately negative. These overlooked foci are usually microinvasive in size but occasionally are larger. Because they lack surrounding myoepithelial cells, they blend into the negative background on immunostains (**Fig. 9**). They also are generally set amid abundant in situ carcinoma with distracting myoepithelial layer positivity. Careful correlation with the morphologic findings on routine sections is critical for ensuring that suspicious foci are adequately evaluated. A matched hematoxylin-and eosin-stained section cut at the same time as the immunohistochemical slides is highly useful, as invasive foci may appear only on the

Fig. 9. Easily overlooked microinvasive tumor (*arrowheads*). This calponin immunostain was misinterpreted as showing no evidence of invasive carcinoma.

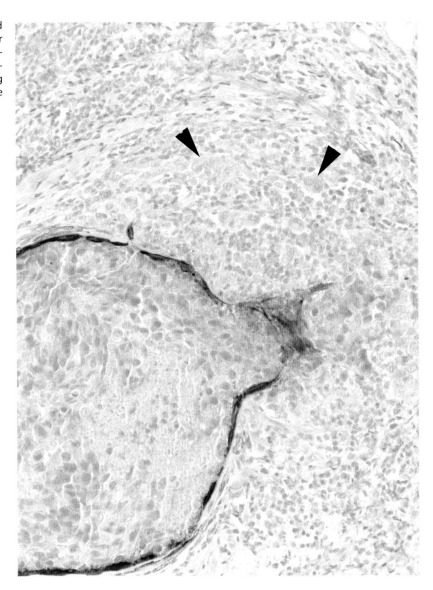

deeper sections. Attention to the possibility of immunonegative epithelial cells in the background is important. Additionally, cytokeratin stains can be invaluable for identifying subtle invasive foci by highlighting the presence of irregularly dispersed epithelial cells (**Fig. 10**). We routinely perform cytokeratin stains in conjunction with the myoepithelial markers to help us recognize these easy-to-miss invasive foci.

MYOEPITHELIAL CELL LAYER ATTENUATION

The normal myoepithelial layer is fairly robust, with numerous myoepithelial cells surrounding the ducts and acini. However, reductions in myoepithelial cell density and the corresponding appearance of gaps in the myoepithelial cell layer are commonly observed in both benign and malignant conditions. The process by which these gaps form and their biologic significance are not well understood. In some cases, the gaps may be generated by mechanical factors: distension of the glandular space by an intraductal proliferation exceeds the rate at which the myoepithelial cells can repopulate the gland. In other cases, the gaps may be the more specific result of signaling from the luminal cells and/or stroma. Intrinsic properties of the myoepithelial

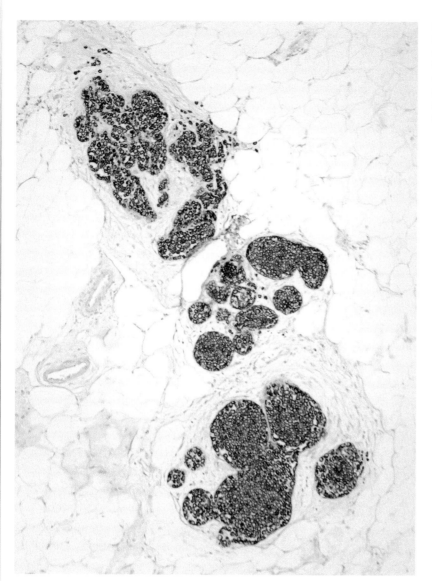

Fig. 10. Invasive and in situ lobular carcinoma. A cytokeratin immunostain highlights the presence of small numbers of infiltrative carcinoma cells percolating into the stroma.

cells likely also govern their density, either as a physiologic or neoplastic phenomenon. These potential mechanisms of myoepithelial cell layer attenuation are not mutually exclusive. The significance of these gaps is not clear, but in the right environment, they may facilitate the development of neoplasia and the progression to invasive carcinoma.[3–6]

It is an obvious but not insignificant problem that the fewer myoepithelial cells there are, the more difficult they are to recognize. This is particularly true on p63 immunostains, where scattered positive nuclei can be quite inconspicuous (**Fig. 11**A). The smooth muscle markers are better at highlighting myoepithelial cells when they are few in number (**Fig. 11**B), because these stains can pick up the elongate cytoplasmic processes. In some examples, small glandular structures may appear completely devoid of myoepithelial cells by p63, but calponin and smooth muscle myosin heavy chain confirm the presence of a few cells. Reliance on p63 alone can lead to a misdiagnosis of invasion in such instances.

Fig. 11. Flat epithelial atypia with attenuated myoepithelial cell layer. (*A*) Several glands appear nearly negative for myoepithelial cells on a p63 immunostain. (*B*) The myoepithelial cells are more readily visualized with a cytoplasmic marker such as smooth muscle myosin heavy chain.

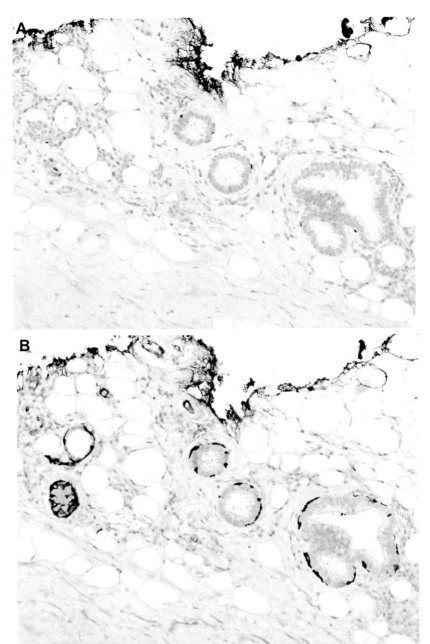

Gaps in the myoepithelial cell layer may be dispersed along the gland perimeter (**Fig. 12**A). Alternatively, there may be an abrupt and total loss of myoepithelial cells next to areas with an intact myoepithelial cell layer (**Fig. 12**B). Whether the latter pattern signifies early or incipient invasion is highly controversial. As long as some myoepithelial cells are identified around a gland profile, it is generally assumed to represent an in situ process. Occasionally, rounded tumor nests lack evidence of myoepithelial cells even when evaluated with multiple markers. This finding should raise concern for invasive carcinoma, especially if there is minimal myoepithelial cell

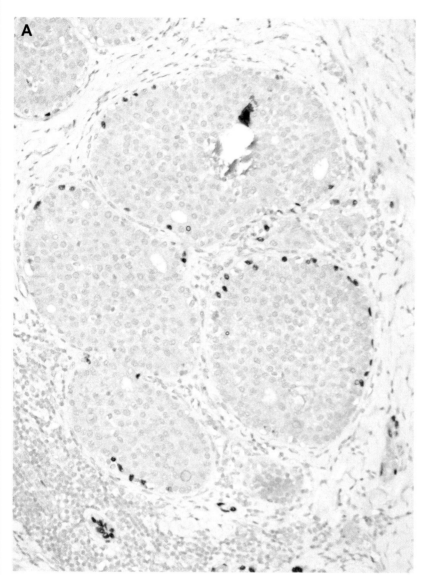

Fig. 12. Two examples of ductal carcinoma in situ with myoepithelial cell attenuation and loss. (*A*) Gaps in the myoepithelial cell layer are distributed around the perimeter of the glands.

layer attenuation in the background. If there is a spectrum of attenuation in the background, more caution is warranted before a diagnosis of invasion is rendered. Careful evaluation of the morphologic features in either setting is essential for determining if the findings represent deceptive invasive carcinoma. If the immuno-negative nests demonstrate a confluent growth pattern, an irregular distribution inconsistent with the branching ductal system, or contour irregularities, a diagnosis of invasion is favored.

Although the issue of myoepithelial cell layer attenuation is most often considered in the context of in situ carcinoma, it also occurs in atypical prolif-erations such as flat epithelial atypia[18] and benign lesions such as radial scars. Up to 12% of radial scars uncomplicated by either carcinoma or atypia show notable myoepithelial cell layer attenuation in either the nidus or the proliferative corona (Warnnissorn M, Koerner FC, and Lerwill MF, in preparation). Loss of myoepithelium around the central distorted tubules may be mistaken for

Fig. 12. (*B*) Abrupt loss of myoepithelial cells next to areas with an intact myoepithelial cell layer. Several nests appear completely negative for myoepithelial cells on a calponin immunostain and should raise concern for invasion.

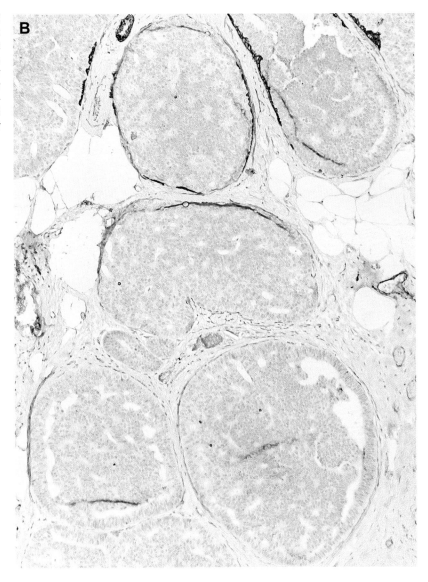

evidence of invasive tubular carcinoma. However, only rarely are there tubules that are entirely negative for myoepithelial cells, and such tubules are morphologically indistinguishable from adjacent ones with intact myoepithelium (**Fig. 13**). An encircling rim of basement membrane is usually still discernible. As expected for a radial scar, the tubules lack cytologic atypia and remain confined to the fibroelastotic stroma of the nidus.[19] Morphology, once again, is the critical determinant.

ABSENCE OF MYOEPITHELIAL CELLS IN BENIGN CONDITIONS

Rare benign conditions may lack myoepithelial cells. Their absence may be artifactual in nature, as occurs with displaced epithelium, or an intrinsic characteristic of the lesion, as with microglandular adenosis.

Epithelial displacement is a recognized phenomenon that can occur after needling or surgical procedures, and is particularly common with

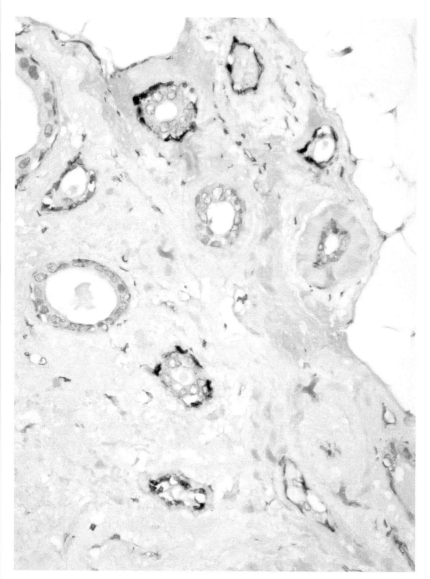

Fig. 13. Radial scar with myoepithelial cell loss around benign glands in the nidus, as demonstrated on a combined p63/smooth muscle actin immunostain.

papillary lesions.[20–23] The displaced epithelium may become dislodged into the stroma or vascular spaces and mimic an invasive process. Myoepithelial cell markers are only sometimes helpful in this setting. If myoepithelial cells are identified, the findings support artifactual displacement. However, epithelium may become dislodged without any accompanying myoepithelial cells. The absence of myoepithelial cells therefore does not constitute evidence of stromal invasion in this context. Several morphologic features can help one to evaluate these foci. If the primary lesion is benign (ie,

a papilloma) and the epithelial clusters have similar benign cytology, then the epithelium is most likely displaced. Displaced epithelium in stroma should be confined to the biopsy site reaction and should not be present in normal stroma. Epithelial clusters within the latter are most consistent with invasive carcinoma. Additionally, displaced epithelial clusters often show degenerative or squamoid changes. Distinguishing displaced epithelium from invasive carcinoma can be particularly challenging in the setting of in situ carcinoma, because the epithelium will have malignant characteristics.

In cases with equivocal findings that are associated with in situ carcinoma, we tend to favor a diagnosis of invasion or at least suspicion for invasion rather than a diagnosis of displaced epithelium.

The absence of myoepithelial cells in microglandular adenosis can be misleading if the characteristic histologic features of the lesion are overlooked.[24–27] In practice, though, the problem is not so much the underdiagnosis of this rare lesion, but its overdiagnosis; we find that most cases in which this diagnosis is considered actually represent conventional invasive carcinomas.

VARIABLE ANTIGENICITY

It should not be assumed that all myoepithelial cells express the same markers, or that their expression is static. The regulation of these markers, the molecular differences between myoepithelial cells in ducts and lobules, and the state of myoepithelial differentiation in various lesions and physiologic conditions all remain poorly understood. Most benign myoepithelial cells are co-reactive for smooth muscle actin, calponin, smooth muscle myosin heavy chain, and p63. Neoplastic myoepithelial cells often show variable reactivity for these markers. Non-neoplastic myoepithelial cells may also demonstrate variable antigenicity on occasion. This can be observed both in the setting of in situ carcinomas (**Fig. 14**) and benign proliferative lesions (**Fig. 15**). In our experience, smooth muscle myosin heavy chain is the antigen whose expression is most often reduced or absent in this circumstance. These observations underscore the fact that more than one myoepithelial marker is needed to corroborate the presence or absence of a myoepithelial cell layer.

PAPILLARY LESIONS

Many pathologists use myoepithelial cell markers to help differentiate between benign and malignant papillary lesions. The general principle is that papillomas have myoepithelial cells along their papillae, whereas papillary carcinomas do not. Although this is generally true, papillary lesions are varied in their nature, and this rule of thumb cannot be followed blindly.

Three different aspects of the myoepithelial cell layer can be considered in papillary lesions. First, the ratio of myoepithelium to epithelium within a lesion can help one to determine whether there is a proliferative epithelial component. Second, the integrity of the myoepithelial cell layer along the epithelial–stromal interface of the papillae can provide some supportive information as to whether a papillary lesion is benign or malignant.

Finally, the integrity of the myoepithelial cell layer along the perimeter of the presumed glandular space is important for differentiating noninvasive from invasive papillary carcinoma. As we consider each of these facets, we will focus mainly on the usefulness of myoepithelial cell markers in diagnosis. For a more detailed discussion of the morphologic features of papillary lesions, the reader is referred to several recent articles,[28–30] including one in this issue of The Clinics.

The intricate three-dimensional architecture of benign papillomas can result in complex glandular patterns that may be mistaken for cribriform ductal carcinoma in situ. Stains for myoepithelial markers can help delineate myoepithelial-covered fibrovascular septae between the glands, revealing that the cribriform-like appearance is due to the aggregation of many individual glands lined by a single layer of ductal cells. Myoepithelial cell markers can thus be used as surrogate markers for intervening stroma. When a papilloma is involved by usual ductal hyperplasia or ductal carcinoma in situ, the proliferative masses of cells lack the stromal septae and their associated myoepithelial cells. Large cellular areas without myoepithelial cells therefore indicate to the observer that a pure epithelial proliferation is present, but this finding does not provide information as to the nature of the proliferation. Evaluation of standard cytologic and architectural features in the proliferative cells is necessary for the determination of benignity or malignancy.[28,31]

Specific evaluation of the myoepithelial cell layer along histologically-identified fibrovascular cores can provide support for a benign or malignant diagnosis. Benign papillomas generally have a robust and continuous myoepithelial cell layer along their stromal cores. When atypical ductal hyperplasia or ductal carcinoma in situ secondarily involves a pre-existing papilloma, the underlying myoepithelial cell layer often becomes attenuated, much as it does when the same processes involve nonpapillomatous ducts. Therefore, loss of myoepithelium may signal a neoplastic process in the overlying epithelium. Two caveats apply. Benign usual ductal hyperplasia may also be associated with a diminished myoepithelial cell layer (Lerwill MF, personal observations), so this feature is not specific to malignancy. Nor is it a sensitive marker of malignancy: just the way many examples of in situ carcinoma have a continuous myoepithelial cell layer, so too may in situ carcinomas that secondarily involve papillomas. The evaluation of epithelial proliferations in pre-existing papillomas should therefore not rest on the amount of underlying myoepithelium, but must be based on the characteristics of the epithelial cells themselves.

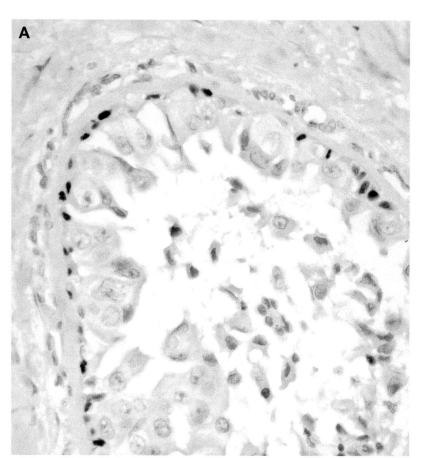

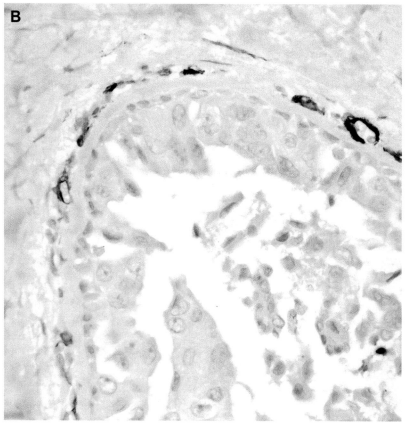

Fig. 14. Ductal carcinoma in situ with variable myoepithelial antigenicity. (*A*) Intact myoepithelial cell layer labeled with p63. (*B*) The myoepithelial cells are negative for smooth muscle myosin heavy chain. Only periductal vascular staining is present.

Fig. 15. Tubular adenosis with variable myoepithelial antigenicity. (*A*) Robust myoepithelial cell layer detected on a calponin immunostain. (*B*) Only weak and patchy reactivity is seen with smooth muscle myosin heavy chain.

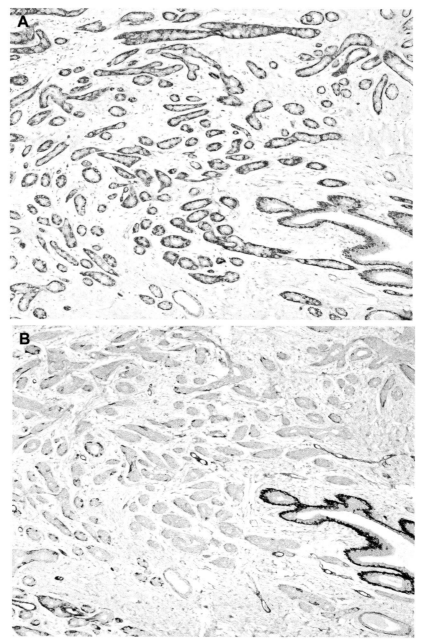

Papillary carcinomas present a somewhat different picture. In these tumors, the papillae are neoplastic and not the result of an in situ carcinoma growing on the scaffolding of a benign papilloma. Papillary carcinomas have thin and delicate papillae, in contrast to the larger and more fibrotic papillae of papillomas. The neoplastic papillae lack myoepithelial cells. In this context, the failure to identify myoepithelial cells on immunohistochemical stains provides secondary evidence of malignancy. However, reliance on the absence of myoepithelial cells for diagnosis is not recommended because it is not always easy to distinguish neoplastic papillae from the nonneoplastic papillae of a papilloma colonized by in situ carcinoma, and the latter is subject to the specificity issues noted above. A diagnosis of malignancy should be fundamentally based on the presence of malignant features in the ductal cells.

Lastly, myoepithelial cell markers are helpful in the distinction of in situ from invasive papillary carcinoma. This is the area where we find the markers most useful in the evaluation of papillary tumors of the breast. Invasive papillary carcinomas frequently mimic large ducts involved by ductal carcinoma in situ (**Fig. 16**) and are commonly mistaken for such. The absence of myoepithelial cells along the perimeter indicates an invasive process. Careful evaluation of the morphologic features will reveal findings inconsistent with an in

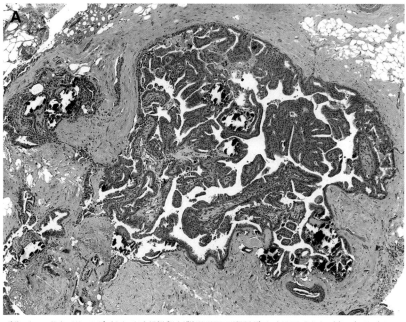

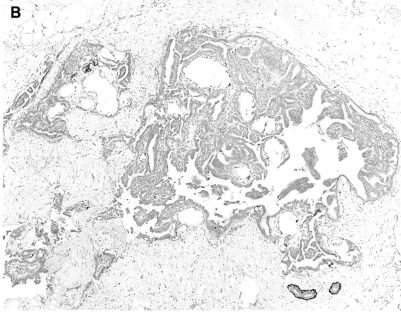

Fig. *16.* (*A*) Invasive papillary carcinoma with irregular borders. (*B*) A p63 immunostain demonstrates a complete lack of myoepithelial cells around the tumor. Two benign ductules with an intact myoepithelial cell layer are located at bottom right.

situ process, including irregular tumor borders, confluent distribution, and engulfment of normal lobules, vessels, fat, and collagenous stroma. Even when the tumor mass appears circumscribed at low-power, high-power evaluation reveals discontinuity along the periphery and the absence of a continuous duct wall. These findings, coupled with the absence of myoepithelium, support a diagnosis of invasive papillary carcinoma.

Two special subtypes of papillary carcinoma warrant comment. Intracystic papillary carcinoma, in which a papillary or polypoid mass grows within a cystically dilated space, has long been assumed to represent a form of ductal carcinoma in situ. Recent studies, however, have revealed a lack of myoepithelial cells around these tumors, suggesting that they may in fact represent relatively indolent invasive carcinomas.[11,32] This would explain the rare examples of metastatic carcinoma developing in cases of intracystic papillary carcinoma.[33] Nevertheless, this group of lesions as a whole has a good prognosis, especially when the tumor is confined to the cystic space, and the term "encapsulated papillary carcinoma" has been suggested to avoid classification as an invasive papillary carcinoma and the risk of overtreatment.[11,32]

Solid papillary carcinoma, a form of ductal carcinoma that often has neuroendocrine differentiation, occurs in both an in situ and invasive form. When invasive, it tends to form large, superficially rounded nests. This bluntly invasive pattern can lead to miscategorization as an in situ carcinoma. Evaluation for myoepithelial cells reveals their absence in many cases of solid papillary carcinoma.[34–37] Even so, many have considered these tumors to be in situ, but the development of metastases that have the same morphology supports that some examples are indeed bluntly invasive neoplasms.[34,36,37] Similar morphologic features as detailed above for invasive papillary carcinoma aid in the recognition of the invasive forms of this tumor.

SPINDLE CELL LESIONS

One additional usage for p63 takes advantage of the fact that it is frequently expressed in mammary spindle cell carcinomas but not in mesenchymal lesions.[38–40] p63 can therefore be used as part of a panel to help evaluate whether a spindle cell neoplasm is of epithelial origin or not, a frequently problematic issue.

SUMMARY

Myoepithelial cell markers can be invaluable for the differentiation of invasive from noninvasive processes in the breast. Their interpretation,

however, can be complicated by patterns of reactivity that may lead one to falsely conclude that a myoepithelial cell layer is present when it is not, and vice versa. Each of the commonly used markers has certain advantages and disadvantages. We therefore suggest the use of at least two markers for complementary interpretation. Our routine "rule-out invasion" panel consists of three myoepithelial markers (calponin, smooth muscle myosin heavy chain, and p63), a cytokeratin immunostain, and a matched hematoxylin- and eosin-stained section.

Myoepithelial markers are also often used in the evaluation of papillary lesions, as malignant papillary lesions commonly have diminished or absent myoepithelium. Although these stains may provide some supportive information, the cytologic and architectural characteristics of the epithelial proliferation are the keys to the diagnosis. We almost never use myoepithelial cell markers to determine whether a papillary proliferation is benign, atypical, or malignant. We do use them, however, to evaluate for possible invasion in malignant papillary tumors, as invasive papillary carcinomas can strikingly mimic in situ lesions.

Awareness of the potential diagnostic pitfalls, evaluation of the morphology of the positively staining cells, and careful correlation with the findings on routine hematoxylin- and eosin-stained sections are the keys to the successful use of myoepithelial cell markers in diagnostic breast pathology.

REFERENCES

1. Emerman JT, Vogl AW. Cell size and shape changes in the myoepithelium of the mammary gland during differentiation. Anat Rec 1986;216(3):405–15.
2. Gudjonsson T, Adriance MC, Sternlicht MD, et al. Myoepithelial cells: their origin and function in breast morphogenesis and neoplasia. J Mammary Gland Biol Neoplasia 2005;10(3):261–72.
3. Hu M, Yao J, Carroll DK, et al. Regulation of in situ to invasive breast carcinoma transition. Cancer Cell 2008;13(5):394–406.
4. Polyak K, Hu M. Do myoepithelial cells hold the key for breast tumor progression? J Mammary Gland Biol Neoplasia 2005;10(3):231–47.
5. Man YG, Tai L, Barner R, et al. Cell clusters overlying focally disrupted mammary myoepithelial cell layers and adjacent cells within the same duct display different immunohistochemical and genetic features: implications for tumor progression and invasion. Breast Cancer Res 2003;5(6):R231–41.
6. Man YG, Zhang Y, Shen T, et al. cDNA expression profiling reveals elevated gene expression in cell

clusters overlying focally disrupted myoepithelial cell layers: implications for breast tumor invasion. Breast Cancer Res Treat 2005;89(2):199–208.

7. Lerwill MF. Current practical applications of diagnostic immunohistochemistry in breast pathology. Am J Surg Pathol 2004;28(8):1076–91.

8. Barbareschi M, Pecciarini L, Cangi MG, et al. p63, a p53 homologue, is a selective nuclear marker of myoepithelial cells of the human breast. Am J Surg Pathol 2001;25(8):1054–60.

9. Werling RW, Hwang H, Yaziji H, et al. Immunohistochemical distinction of invasive from noninvasive breast lesions: a comparative study of p63 versus calponin and smooth muscle myosin heavy chain. Am J Surg Pathol 2003;27(1):82–90.

10. Ribeiro-Silva A, Zambelli Ramalho LN, Britto Garcia S, et al. The relationship between p63 and p53 expression in normal and neoplastic breast tissue. Arch Pathol Lab Med 2003;127(3):336–40.

11. Collins LC, Carlo VP, Hwang H, et al. Intracystic papillary carcinomas of the breast: a reevaluation using a panel of myoepithelial cell markers. Am J Surg Pathol 2006;30(8):1002–7.

12. Moritani S, Kushima R, Sugihara H, et al. Availability of CD10 immunohistochemistry as a marker of breast myoepithelial cells on paraffin sections. Mod Pathol 2002;15(4):397–405.

13. Heatley M, Maxwell P, Whiteside C, et al. Cytokeratin intermediate filament expression in benign and malignant breast disease. J Clin Pathol 1995;48(1):26–32.

14. Gillett CE, Bobrow LG, Millis RR. S100 protein in human mammary tissue–immunoreactivity in breast carcinoma, including Paget's disease of the nipple, and value as a marker of myoepithelial cells. J Pathol 1990;160(1):19–24.

15. Zhang RR, Man YG, Vang R, et al. A subset of morphologically distinct mammary myoepithelial cells lacks corresponding immunophenotypic markers. Breast Cancer Res 2003;5(5):R151–6.

16. Kovacs A, Walker RA. P-cadherin as a marker in the differential diagnosis of breast lesions. J Clin Pathol 2003;56(2):139–41.

17. Rabban JT, Chen YY. D2-40 expression by breast myoepithelium: potential pitfalls in distinguishing intralymphatic carcinoma from in situ carcinoma. Hum Pathol 2008;39(2):175–83.

18. Lerwill MF. Flat epithelial atypia of the breast. Arch Pathol Lab Med 2008;132(4):615–21.

19. Rabban JT, Sgroi DC. Sclerosing lesions of the breast. Semin Diagn Pathol 2004;21(1):42–7.

20. Youngson BJ, Cranor M, Rosen PP. Epithelial displacement in surgical breast specimens following needling procedures. Am J Surg Pathol 1994;18(9):896–903.

21. Youngson BJ, Liberman L, Rosen PP. Displacement of carcinomatous epithelium in surgical breast specimens following stereotaxic core biopsy. Am J Clin Pathol 1995;103(5):598–602.

22. Douglas-Jones AG, Verghese A. Diagnostic difficulty arising from displaced epithelium after core biopsy in intracystic papillary lesions of the breast. J Clin Pathol 2002;55(10):780–3.

23. Nagi C, Bleiweiss I, Jaffer S. Epithelial displacement in breast lesions: a papillary phenomenon. Arch Pathol Lab Med 2005;129(11):1465–9.

24. Rosen PP. Microglandular adenosis. A benign lesion simulating invasive mammary carcinoma. Am J Surg Pathol 1983;7(2):137–44.

25. Tavassoli FA, Norris HJ. Microglandular adenosis of the breast. A clinicopathologic study of 11 cases with ultrastructural observations. Am J Surg Pathol 1983;7(8):731–7.

26. Clement PB, Azzopardi JG. Microglandular adenosis of the breast – a lesion simulating tubular carcinoma. Histopathology 1983;7(2):169–80.

27. Khalifeh IM, Albarracin C, Diaz LK, et al. Clinical, histopathologic, and immunohistochemical features of microglandular adenosis and transition into in situ and invasive carcinoma. Am J Surg Pathol 2008;32(4):544–52.

28. Oyama T, Koerner FC. Noninvasive papillary proliferations. Semin Diagn Pathol 2004;21(1):32–41.

29. Mulligan AM, O'Malley FP. Papillary lesions of the breast: a review. Adv Anat Pathol 2007;14(2):108–19.

30. Collins LC, Schnitt SJ. Papillary lesions of the breast: selected diagnostic and management issues. Histopathology 2008;52(1):20–9.

31. Koerner FC. Epithelial proliferations of ductal type. Semin Diagn Pathol 2004;21(1):10–7.

32. Hill CB, Yeh IT. Myoepithelial cell staining patterns of papillary breast lesions: from intraductal papillomas to invasive papillary carcinomas. Am J Clin Pathol 2005;123(1):36–44.

33. Mulligan AM, O'Malley FP. Metastatic potential of encapsulated (intracystic) papillary carcinoma of the breast: a report of 2 cases with axillary lymph node micrometastases. Int J Surg Pathol 2007;15(2):143–7.

34. Maluf HM, Koerner FC. Solid papillary carcinoma of the breast. A form of intraductal carcinoma with endocrine differentiation frequently associated with mucinous carcinoma. Am J Surg Pathol 1995;19(11):1237–44.

35. Dickersin GR, Maluf HM, Koerner FC. Solid papillary carcinoma of breast: an ultrastructural study. Ultrastruct Pathol 1997;21(2):153–61.

36. Nassar H, Qureshi H, Volkanadsay N, et al. Clinicopathologic analysis of solid papillary carcinoma of the breast and associated invasive carcinomas. Am J Surg Pathol 2006;30(4):501–7.

37. Nicolas MM, Wu Y, Middleton LP, et al. Loss of myoepithelium is variable in solid papillary

carcinoma of the breast. Histopathology 2007;
51(5):657–65.

38. Reis-Filho JS, Milanezi F, Paredes J, et al. Novel and
classic myoepithelial/stem cell markers in metaplastic carcinomas of the breast. Appl Immunohistochem Mol Morphol 2003;11(1):1–8.

39. Carter MR, Hornick JL, Lester S, et al. Spindle cell
(sarcomatoid) carcinoma of the breast:

a clinicopathologic and immunohistochemical analysis of 29 cases. Am J Surg Pathol 2006;30(3):
300–9.

40. Cates JM, Dupont WD, Barnes JW, et al. Markers of
epithelial-mesenchymal transition and epithelial
differentiation in sarcomatoid carcinoma: utility in
the differential diagnosis with sarcoma. Appl Immunohistochem Mol Morphol 2008;16(3):251–62.

SPINDLE CELL LESIONS OF THE BREAST

Stuart J. Schnitt, MD

KEYWORDS

• Spindle cell carcinoma • Fibromatosis • Myofibroblastoma • Nodular fasciitis • Breast

ABSTRACT

S pindle cell lesions of the breast represent a heterogeneous group of reactive and neoplastic disorders that commonly present diagnostic challenges. Arguably, the most important of these lesions to recognize is spindle cell carcinoma, a type of metaplastic carcinoma. This review focuses on those spindle cell lesions of the breast that are most likely to be encountered in clinical practice or that produce particular diagnostic difficulties.

SPINDLE CELL LESIONS OF THE BREAST

OVERVIEW

A variety of reactive and neoplastic lesions of the breast are characterized by a proliferation of spindle cells.[1–4] Because these lesions are uncommon, many surgical pathologists, even those who have considerable experience, often find them diagnostically challenging.

When any spindle cell lesion is encountered in the breast, the diagnosis of spindle cell carcinoma (a type of metaplastic carcinoma) should always be given serious consideration, and that diagnosis should not be dismissed unless there is histologic or immunophenotypic evidence to exclude it. The possibility of a phyllodes tumor should also be considered because the epithelial component may be difficult to identify in some cases, particularly in cases of malignant lesions characterized by prominent stromal overgrowth or in cases with small biopsy samples. In fact, the definitive categorization of any spindle cell lesion of the breast may be difficult or impossible to determine in the limited sampling afforded by core needle biopsy, and a cautious approach to the diagnosis of spindle cell lesions in needle biopsy specimens is prudent.

Many spindle cell lesions that occur in other anatomic sites (such as neural tumors and smooth muscle tumors) may also be seen in the breast. This review focuses on those lesions that are most likely to be encountered in clinical practice or that produce particular diagnostic difficulties.

SPINDLE CELL CARCINOMA

OVERVIEW

Some carcinomas of the breast that are included within the broader category of metaplastic carcinoma are composed of a pure or predominant population of spindle cells. Tumors of this type have been designated as metaplastic carcinoma, sarcomatoid carcinoma, spindle cell metaplastic carcinoma, and spindle cell carcinoma.[1–8] Spindle

> ### Key Features
> #### SPINDLE CELL LESIONS OF THE BREAST
>
> • A diverse group of reactive and neoplastic disorders.
>
> • Correct classification requires a careful histologic assessment of the growth pattern and cytologic features of the spindle cells; the use of adjunctive immunostains may be necessary in some cases.
>
> • A definitive diagnosis may be difficult or impossible in core needle biopsy material.
>
> • Always consider the possibility of spindle cell (metaplastic) carcinoma, regardless of the appearance of the spindle cells.

Department of Pathology, Beth Israel Deaconess Medical Center, Harvard Medical School, 330 Brookline Avenue, Boston, MA 02215, USA
E-mail address: sschnitt@bidmc.harvard.edu

Surgical Pathology 2 (2009) 375–390
doi:10.1016/j.path.2009.02.009

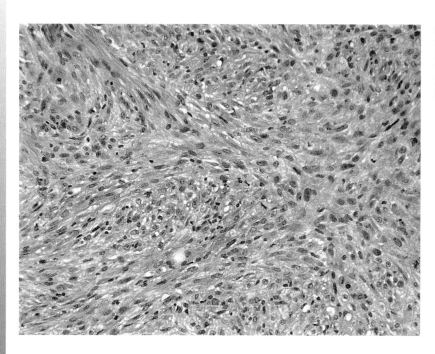

Fig. 1. Spindle cell carcinoma. This lesion is characterized by interlacing fascicles of spindle cells. A mitotic figure is present in one of the cells.

cell carcinomas are uncommon, accounting for less than 1% of invasive breast cancers.

GROSS FEATURES

On gross examination, the tumors are most often gray or white, firm masses that may have an infiltrative appearance. Not infrequently, however, these tumors are grossly circumscribed.

MICROSCOPIC FEATURES

The cells that compose spindle cell carcinomas can vary in appearance from cytologically bland to highly pleomorphic. The growth pattern may be fascicular, fasciitis-like, storiform, or haphazard (**Figs. 1** and **2**). Areas suggestive of vascular spaces are seen in some cases (**Fig. 3**). The mitotic rate is highly variable. The borders of the lesion are

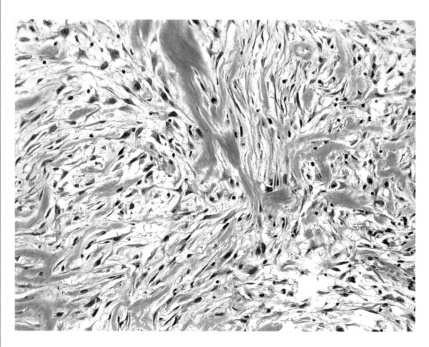

Fig. 2. Spindle cell carcinoma. This spindle cell carcinoma has a fasciitis-like appearance, with spindle and stellate-shaped cells in a partially myxoid stroma.

Fig. 3. Spindle cell carcinoma with pseudovascular spaces.

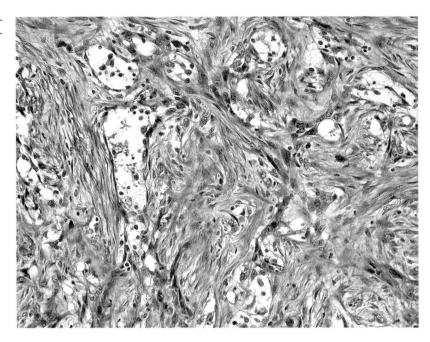

usually infiltrative, with entrapment of mammary ducts and lobules, but some cases exhibit pushing margins. Higher-grade lesions tend to obliterate the normal breast architecture. In some cases, the spindle cells aggregate into small clusters that exhibit a more epithelioid appearance or merge with an overt epithelial component. Areas of squamous differentiation are not infrequent (**Fig. 4**), and

foci of heterologous chondroid or osseous differentiation may be seen. In highly cellular lesions, the stroma between the spindle cells may be inapparent; at the other end of the spectrum, the spindle cells are more widely dispersed in an abundant, collagenized stroma with a keloid-like appearance.

Areas of conventional types of invasive breast carcinoma or ductal carcinoma in situ (DCIS) may

Fig. 4. Spindle cell carcinoma with foci of squamous differentiation.

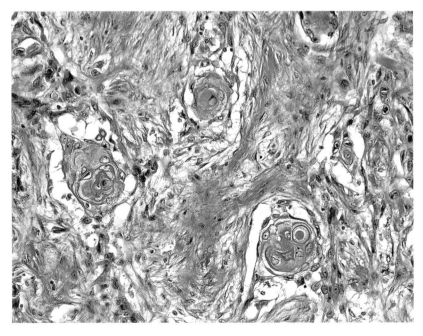

be seen in association with the spindle cell component, and when present, these lesions can provide useful clues to the epithelial nature of the tumor (**Fig. 5**). However, in pure spindle cell carcinomas without associated overt epithelial foci or associated DCIS, the use of immunohistochemical stains for cytokeratin may be required to arrive at the correct diagnosis. It should be noted however, that cytokeratin immunoreactivity may be focal and that the use of a panel of anticytokeratin antibodies may be required to demonstrate cytokeratin positivity. Broad spectrum cytokeratin antibodies (such as antibody MNF116) and antibodies to high-molecular-weight/basal cytokeratins (such as antibody 34βE12 or antibodies to cytokeratin 5/6) are the most sensitive for the detection of cytokeratin expression in this setting.[8] In contrast, stains with antibodies such as CAM 5.2 and AE1/AE3 are often either negative or only focally positive (**Fig. 6**). The neoplastic cells also commonly express vimentin, smooth muscle actin, muscle-specific actin, and particularly, p63 (**Fig. 7**). Expression by these tumors of actins, p63, basal cytokeratins, and other markers commonly associated with myoepithelial cells has been used as evidence supporting a myoepithelial or basal phenotype for many of these tumors.[9–11] Indeed, the distinction between spindle cell carcinomas and lesions previously described as myoepithelial carcinomas/malignant myoepitheliomas is probably just one of semantics. Spindle cell carcinomas are typically negative for estrogen receptor and progesterone receptor expression and for HER2 protein

Da Ko

overexpression and gene amplification (ie, "triple negative").

One type of spindle cell carcinoma worthy of particular note is the low-grade, fibromatosis-like,

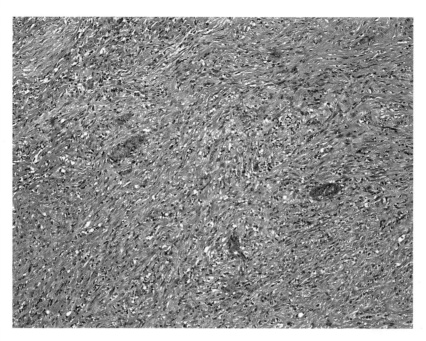

> **△△ *Differential Diagnosis***
> Spindle Cell Lesions of the Breast
>
> *Bland spindle cells*
>
> - Scars
> - Fibromatosis
> - Myofibroblastoma
> - Pseudoangiomatous stromal hyperplasia (fascicular type)
> - Adenomyoepithelioma
> - Spindle cell (metaplastic) carcinoma
>
> *Atypical spindle cells*
>
> - Spindle cell (metaplastic) carcinoma
> - Malignant phyllodes tumor
> - Nodular fasciitis
> - Primary sarcoma
> - Metastatic sarcoma
> - Metastatic spindle cell (sarcomatoid) carcinoma
> - Metastatic malignant melanoma

Fig. 5. Spindle cell carcinoma with overt epithelial differentiation. Several islands of epithelial cells with glandular lumina are present among the spindle cells.

Fig. 6. Spindle cell carcinoma. (*A*) In this immunostain using anticytokeratin antibodies AE1/AE3, the epithelial cells of the benign mammary ducts show strong cytokeratin expression, but most of the cells that compose the spindle cell carcinoma are cytokeratin-negative. (*B*) In contrast, this MNF116 immunostain of the same lesion demonstrates strong cytokeratin expression in many of the spindle cells.

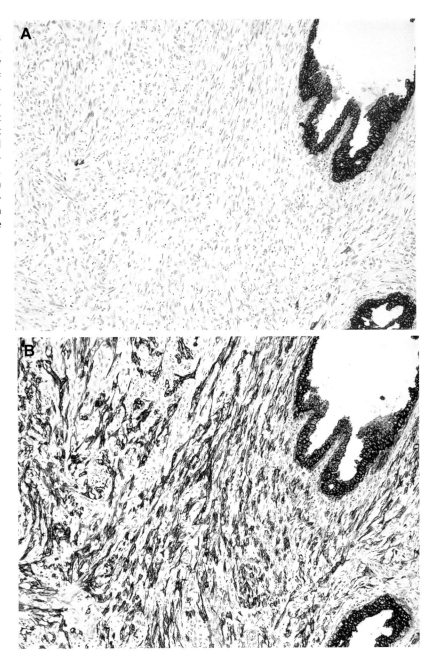

metaplastic carcinoma.[12,13] These lesions, which may arise either de novo or in association with papillomas and benign sclerosing lesions,[14] are composed of bland spindle cells resembling those seen in scars or fibromatosis (**Fig. 8**). In contrast to the cells of scars or fibromatosis, however, the spindle cells that compose these lesions show expression of cytokeratin, and in some cases show epithelioid cell clusters or small foci of squamous differentiation.

DIFFERENTIAL DIAGNOSIS

Given the wide range of appearances of spindle cell carcinoma, the differential diagnosis is broad and includes the other spindle cell lesions

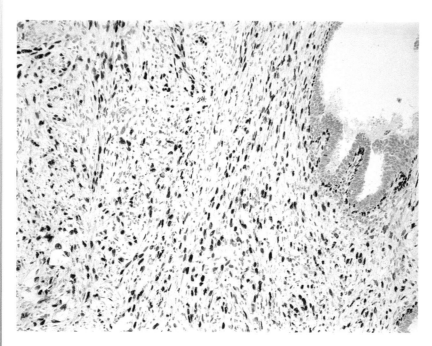

Fig. 7. Spindle cell carcinoma immunostained for p63. Many of the tumor cells show nuclear expression of p63.

discussed in this article as well as malignant phyllodes tumors with prominent stromal overgrowth. It is important to note that a malignant spindle cell tumor of the breast is much more likely to be a spindle cell carcinoma or a malignant phyllodes tumor than a sarcoma. As noted previously in this article, the presence of areas of overt epithelial differentiation or associated DCIS is a valuable clue to the diagnosis of spindle cell carcinoma. In cases without such features, the demonstration of cytokeratin expression by the neoplastic cells may be required to arrive at the correct diagnosis.

DIAGNOSIS

The diagnosis of spindle cell carcinoma can be problematic in breast excision specimens and can be even more difficult in core needle biopsy specimens. Highly atypical and cellular lesions may initially lead to the erroneous impression of a sarcoma. At the other end of the spectrum, cytologically bland, paucicellular lesions may be misidentified as a scar or fibromatosis. The best way to avoid missing a diagnosis of spindle cell carcinoma is to always consider it as a diagnostic possibility whenever a spindle cell lesion is encountered in a breast biopsy and to have a low threshold for performing immunostains for cytokeratins and p63 when such lesions are encountered. However, the definitive classification of a spindle cell lesion may not be possible using

core needle biopsy samples, and in such cases the final diagnosis should await the surgical excision specimen.

PROGNOSIS

Spindle cell carcinomas are less frequently associated with axillary lymph node metastases than are conventional types of invasive breast cancer.[4] Recent studies suggest a poorer prognosis for spindle cell carcinomas than for conventional mammary carcinomas,[8] and it has been suggested that the clinical behavior of spindle cell carcinomas, particularly those that lack or have a minimal recognizable epithelial component, is more akin to that of sarcomas than carcinomas.[7]

Fibromatosis-like metaplastic carcinomas have been reported to be associated with a high rate of local recurrence. Although no instances of metastasis were observed in the initial report of these cases,[12] regional and distant metastases have subsequently been reported in a small proportion of patients who have these lesions.[13]

FIBROMATOSIS

OVERVIEW

Mammary fibromatosis is an infiltrative, locally aggressive proliferation of fibroblasts and myofibroblasts that typically presents as a firm mass that may be mistaken for carcinoma clinically

Fig. 8. Low-grade, fibromatosis-like metaplastic carcinoma. (*A*) Medium-power image shows a haphazard proliferation of spindle cells in a collagenized stroma. The lesion is infiltrating adipose tissue. (*B*) High-power view demonstrates the bland cytologic features of the spindle cells.

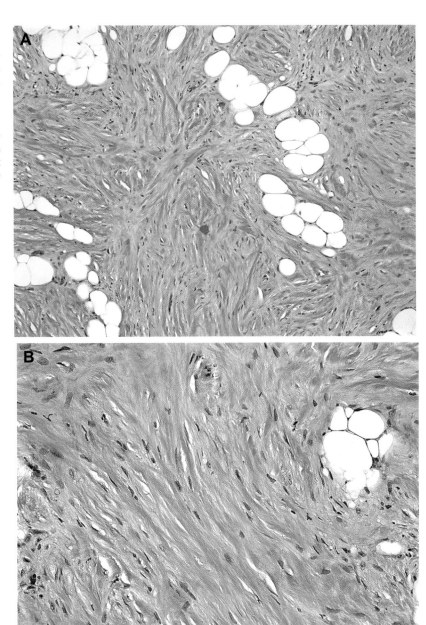

and mammographically. Most cases are sporadic, but mammary fibromatosis may be seen in association with familial adenomatous polyposis, with Gardner syndrome, or as part of a hereditary desmoid syndrome.[2,15,16]

GROSS FEATURES

On gross examination, fibromatosis most often has a poorly defined or stellate, gray-white-to-tan appearance.

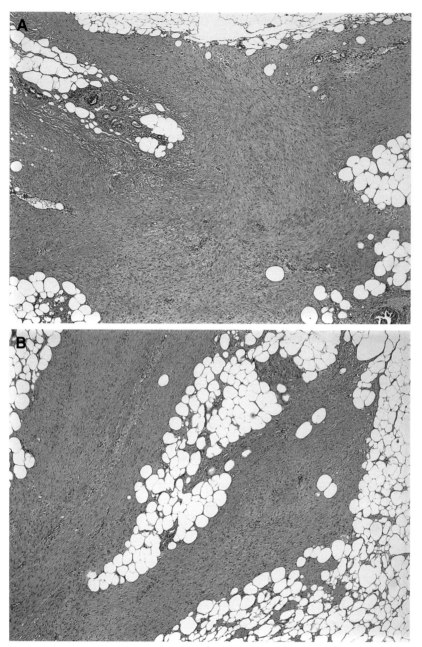

Fig. 9. Fibromatosis. (*A*) Low-power view demonstrates sweeping fascicles of spindle cells surrounding and entrapping normal mammary glandular structures and extending into adipose tissue. (*B*) Another example of fibromatosis with long fascicles of spindle cells extending irregularly into adipose tissue.

MICROSCOPIC FEATURES

The histologic features of mammary fibromatosis are similar to those of desmoid-type fibromatoses in other sites. Uniform, cytologically bland spindle cells with pale eosinophilic cytoplasm, poorly defined cell borders, and oval-to-elongated and tapering nuclei infiltrate the stroma in long, sweeping fascicles, surrounding and entrapping mammary ducts and lobules and extending irregularly into adipose tissue (**Fig. 9**). Mitotic figures are usually not present but may be seen and may even be numerous in focal areas. The cellularity is variable, as is the amount of stromal

Fig. 9. (C) High-power view illustrates the cytologically bland, uniform-appearing spindle cells with indistinct cell borders and tapering nuclei.

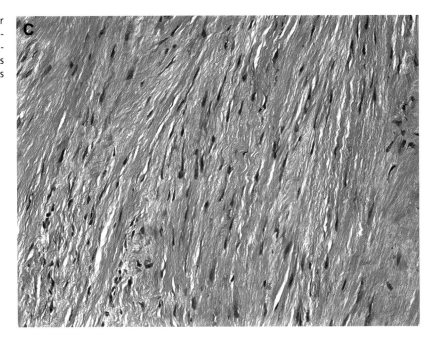

collagen. Cases with abundant stromal collagen have a keloidal appearance. At the other extreme, the stroma may show prominent myxoid change, similar to that seen in nodular fasciitis. Lesions are often more cellular at the periphery than in the center. Lymphoid infiltrates are commonly present and are most prominent at the edges of the lesion.

The spindle cells in cases of fibromatosis show immunostaining for actin; desmin and S100 protein expression can also be seen, but usually in only a minority of cells.[2] Nuclear expression of β-catenin is seen in about three quarters of the cases, and this may be a particularly useful diagnostic adjunct.[17] However, nuclear β-catenin expression is not specific for fibromatosis and may be seen in a small proportion of spindle cell carcinomas and in fibroadenomas and phyllodes tumors.[4]

DIFFERENTIAL DIAGNOSIS

The two lesions that most commonly enter into the differential diagnosis of fibromatosis are scarring from prior trauma (including surgery) and fibromatosis-like metaplastic carcinoma. The presence of hemosiderin deposition, fat necrosis, histiocytes, and foreign body giant cells, and the absence of long fascicles and entrapment of breast ducts and lobules at the periphery favor a diagnosis of scarring. However, in patients who have fibromatosis and who have had prior surgery, it may be difficult or impossible to distinguish areas of postsurgical scarring from residual fibromatosis, and this may create particular problems in the assessment of the excision margins.

Arguably, the most important differential diagnostic consideration is a fibromatosis-like metaplastic carcinoma because these lesions are by definition deceptively bland.[12,13] Useful clues to the diagnosis of fibromatosis-like metaplastic carcinomas include foci in which the cells have an epithelioid appearance and the presence of cytokeratin expression by the spindle cells, although the latter may be difficult to demonstrate and may require the use of several different anticytokeratin antibodies.

Other lesions that may enter into the differential diagnosis of fibromatosis are nodular fasciitis and spindle cell sarcomas. Features useful in distinguishing nodular fasciitis from fibromatosis are discussed later in the article. Sarcomas are usually more cellular than fibromatosis and show nuclear pleomorphism and mitotic activity, including atypical mitoses.

DIAGNOSIS

Although the diagnosis of fibromatosis may be suggested on a core needle biopsy, it may be difficult or impossible to distinguish fibromatosis from a scar or from spindle cell carcinoma in limited tissue samples. Therefore, excision is typically required for a definitive diagnosis.

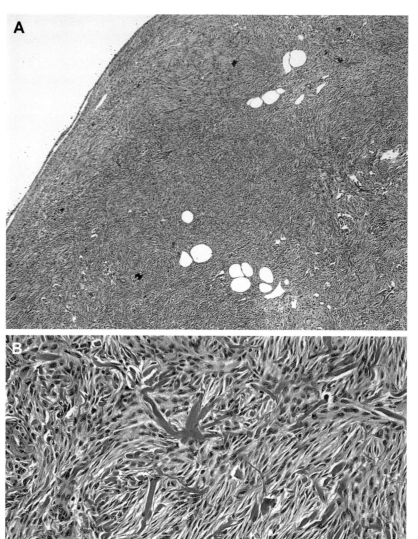

Fig.10. Myofibroblastoma, classic type. (*A*) Low-power view shows a circumscribed lesion composed of spindle cells, collagen, and foci of adipose tissue. (*B*) Higher-power view shows short fascicles of cytologically bland spindle cells and bands of hyalinized collagen.

PROGNOSIS

The major clinical concern for patients who have fibromatosis is local recurrence, which has been reported in approximately 20% to 25% of cases. Recurrences are most common within the first three years after diagnosis.[4] Wide local excision is considered the treatment of choice for patients who have fibromatosis. However, it should be noted that the correlation between margin status and local recurrence is not absolute; some patients with positive margins do not develop local recurrences, and conversely, local recurrences may be seen in patients with negative margins. In addition, there are no histologic features that can be used to reliably predict which lesions are likely to recur locally.

Fig.11. Myofibroblastoma, epithelioid variant. (*A*) Clusters and strands of epithelioid cells are present within a dense collagenous stroma. (*B*) At high power, the epithelioid nature of the cells is even more apparent. The pattern mimics the appearance of an invasive lobular carcinoma.

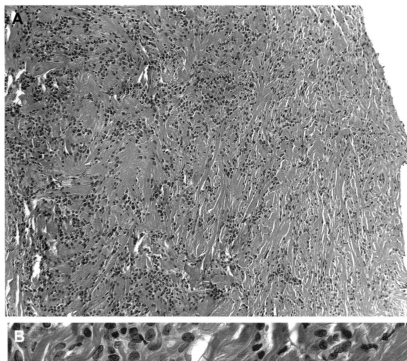

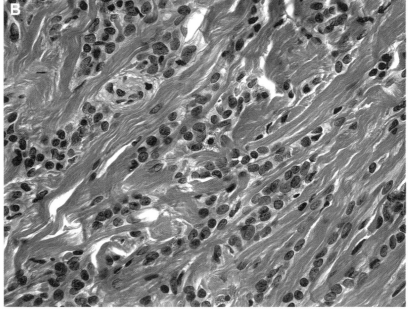

MYOFIBROBLASTOMA

OVERVIEW

Myofibroblastomas are uncommon benign tumors of the breast. Early reports suggested that these lesions occurred more frequently in men than women. However, myofibroblastomas have been identified with increased frequency on screening mammography, and they now appear to occur with equal frequency in women and men.[2,18,20]

These lesions are typically slow growing, circumscribed, mobile masses that are usually mistaken for fibroadenomas on physical examination and mammographic examination.

GROSS FEATURES

Gross examination reveals a lobulated, rubbery, firm nodule with a bulging, homogenous, gray-to-pink, whorled, cut surface.

MICROSCOPIC FEATURES

A variety of patterns may be seen on histologic examination. In the classic type of myofibroblastoma, the tumor is circumscribed but does not have a true capsule. The spindle cells composing the lesion are uniform in appearance, have bland oval nuclei, and are arranged as short fascicles admixed with bands of hyalinized collagen. Mitoses are usually not observed. Variable amounts of fat are typically present within the lesion, as are mast cells and patchy perivascular lymphoplasmacytic infiltrates (**Fig. 10**). The stroma may show myxoid change, smooth muscle differentiation, or chondroid metaplasia. Several variants of myofibroblastoma have been described. The collagenized variant features abundant stromal collagen and little cellularity, whereas in the cellular variant, the ratio of cells to stroma is higher than in the classic type. An infiltrative variant has been described in which the tumor margins are irregular. Cases with nuclear pleomorphism have also been reported (atypical myofibroblastoma), but cytologic atypia in this setting does not seem to have clinical importance. In the myxoid variant, stromal myxoid change is particularly

prominent. Finally, some myofibroblastomas are composed partially or predominantly of cells with an epithelioid appearance that are arranged in cords, alveolar groups, and linear strands. When this pattern predominates, the histologic features may raise concern for an invasive carcinoma, particularly invasive lobular carcinoma (**Fig. 11**).

The cells of myofibroblastomas typically show expression of CD34 and desmin, with more variable positivity for actin. Expression of estrogen and progesterone receptors and bcl2 is common.[2,21] Expression of estrogen and progesterone receptors in an epithelioid myofibroblastoma may compound the confusion of this type of cancer with invasive carcinoma.

DIFFERENTIAL DIAGNOSIS

Given the variable appearance of myofibroblastoma, it should not be surprising that the differential diagnosis is broad and includes a variety of reactive and benign spindle cell lesions, spindle cell sarcoma, and carcinoma (**Table 1**). A few of these are worthy of particular note. The histologic features of myofibroblastoma overlap with those of spindle cell lipoma. Furthermore, these two tumors share genetic abnormalities, suggesting a close relationship between them.[21,22] Pseudoangiomatous stromal hyperplasia (PASH) may exhibit foci of increased cellularity with a fascicular arrangement of myofibroblasts that produces a myofibroblastoma-like appearance. This suggests that PASH and myofibroblastomas represent two ends of a spectrum of myofibroblastic lesions. As with other spindle

---

Table 1
Lesions to consider in the differential diagnosis of myofibroblastoma

Reactive and benign spindle cell lesions
- ○ Nodular fasciitis
- ○ Solitary fibrous tumor
- ○ Spindle cell lipoma
- ○ Peripheral nerve sheath tumors
- ○ Smooth muscle tumors
- ○ Fascicular pseudoangiomatous stromal hyperplasia

Spindle cell sarcomas

Carcinomas
- ○ Spindle cell (metaplastic) carcinoma
- ○ Other types of carcinoma (particularly invasive lobular carcinoma, which can be mimicked by the epithelioid variant of myofibroblastoma)

Fig. 12. Nodular fasciitis. (A) Medium-power view shows spindle cells in a myxoid stroma and foci of erythrocyte extravasation. (B) High-power view shows the tissue culture appearance of the spindle cells, which have vesicular nuclei and variably prominent nucleoli. A mitotic figure is evident.

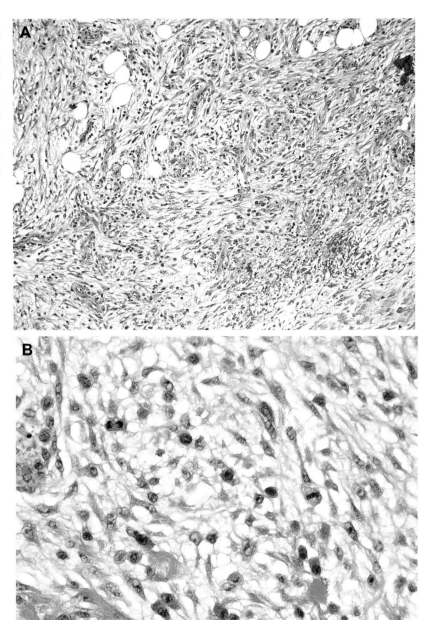

cell lesions, spindle cell carcinoma should be given consideration in the differential diagnosis.

DIAGNOSIS

The diagnosis of myofibroblastoma can be suggested in core needle biopsy samples if the characteristic histologic features are present and the clinical or imaging findings are consistent with that diagnosis. However, as with other spindle cell lesions of the breast, care should be taken to avoid making a definitive diagnosis using core needle biopsy samples unless the findings are unequivocal.

PROGNOSIS

Myofibroblastomas are benign and can be adequately treated with local excision. No instances of local recurrence have been reported.

NODULAR FASCIITIS

OVERVIEW

Nodular fasciitis is uncommonly seen in the breast but is particularly important to recognize because it may mimic a malignant tumor clinically and on radiographic and histologic examination.[2] Lesions of nodular fasciitis may occur either in the subcutaneous tissue of the breast or in the mammary parenchyma. As it does at other sites, nodular fasciitis in the breast presents as a rapidly growing mass that may be painful or tender and that disappears spontaneously within a few months.

GROSS FEATURES

The gross appearance of nodular fasciitis varies with the amount of myxoid stroma and collagen in the lesion, and with its cellularity. Lesions that are more myxoid have a soft, gelatinous cut surface, whereas in lesions that are more collagenized, the cut surface is firm and fibrotic. Most lesions are generally well circumscribed but unencapsulated.[23]

MICROSCOPIC FEATURES

The histologic features of nodular fasciitis in the breast are identical to those of nodular fasciitis elsewhere. The lesion is generally well circumscribed but not encapsulated, and it is composed of plump spindle cells arranged in short fascicles and whorls. The nuclei have prominent nucleoli, but are uniform in appearance. Mitotic figures are readily identifiable and may be numerous. The appearance of these spindle cells (which are fibroblasts and myofibroblasts) has been likened to that of fibroblasts grown in tissue culture. The stroma is typically loose and myxoid and may show cystic change. Extravasated erythrocytes and patchy lymphoid infiltrates are common features (**Fig. 12**). Lymphoid aggregates may be present, especially at the periphery of the lesion. The cellularity of the lesions varies; early lesions are highly cellular, whereas regressing lesions show less cellularity and more stromal collagen deposition. Mammary ducts and lobules are usually not present within the lesion. The myofibroblasts within nodular fasciitis typically express actin, but

this may be focal. Desmin expression is also occasionally seen.

DIFFERENTIAL DIAGNOSIS

The major differential diagnostic considerations are malignant spindle cell tumors (including spindle cell carcinomas and sarcomas) and fibromatosis. Nodular fasciitis lacks the nuclear atypia of sarcomas and most spindle cell carcinomas and does not have the long, sweeping fascicles and infiltrative edge of fibromatosis. Furthermore, in contrast with spindle cell carcinomas, the cells of nodular fasciitis lack cytokeratin expression.

DIAGNOSIS

Given that other spindle cell lesions of the breast (including spindle cell carcinoma and fibromatosis) can have a fasciitis-like appearance, making the correct diagnosis of nodular fasciitis requires adequate tissue sampling, and this may not be possible in the limited material provided by core needle biopsy. Therefore, a definitive diagnosis of nodular fasciitis usually requires using excisional biopsy specimens.

PROGNOSIS

Although nodular fasciitis will spontaneously regress, the clinical presentation of growing mass

---

Pitfalls
POSSIBLE PITFALLS IN THE DIAGNOSIS OF SPINDLE CELL LESIONS OF THE BREAST

! A malignant spindle cell tumor in the breast is more likely to represent a spindle cell carcinoma or the stromal component of a malignant phyllodes tumor than a primary breast sarcoma. Therefore, the diagnosis of primary breast sarcoma should never be made before excluding these other possibilities.

! Some spindle cell carcinomas may be deceptively bland and may resemble a fibromatosis or a scar.

! Cytokeratin staining in spindle cell carcinomas may be focal and may require a panel of anticytokeratin antibodies for its demonstration; broad spectrum anticytokeratin antibodies (such as antibody MNF116) and antibodies to high molecular weight/basal cytokeratins (such as antibody 34βE12 or antibodies to cytokeratin 5/6) are the most sensitive in this setting.

in the breast virtually always prompts a biopsy or excision. Local excision is adequate treatment.

SPINDLE CELL SARCOMAS

OVERVIEW

When a spindle cell sarcoma is identified in the breast, it is more likely to represent the stromal component of a malignant phyllodes tumor than a pure sarcoma. Therefore, the histologic identification of a spindle cell sarcoma should prompt careful evaluation of the lesion for the presence of a benign epithelial component, which, in turn, will lead to the diagnosis of malignant phyllodes tumor.

Among the pure sarcomas of the breast, the most common is angiosarcoma. Other types of sarcoma may also rarely be seen. In addition, sarcomas from other sites may rarely metastasize to the breast.

OTHER LESIONS WITH SPINDLE CELL MORPHOLOGY

In some adenomyoepitheliomas, the myoepithelial cells have a predominantly or exclusively spindle cell appearance. In addition, in some cases of PASH, myofibroblastic proliferation is prominent and may resemble areas seen in myofibroblastoma (fascicular PASH). Finally, some nonsarcomatous, malignant tumors that are metastatic to the breast, such as sarcomatoid renal cell carcinoma and malignant melanoma, may have a spindle cell appearance.

REFERENCES

1. Al-Nafussi A. Spindle cell tumours of the breast: practical approach to diagnosis. Histopathology 1999;35(1):1–13.
2. McMenamin ME, DeSchryver K, Fletcher CD. Fibrous lesions of the breast: a review. Int J Surg Pathol 2000;8(2):99–108.
3. Tse GM, Tan PH, Lui PC, et al. Spindle cell lesions of the breast—the pathologic differential diagnosis. Breast Cancer Res Treat 2007.
4. Lee AH. Recent developments in the histological diagnosis of spindle cell carcinoma, fibromatosis and phyllodes tumour of the breast. Histopathology 2008;52(1):45–57.
5. Wargotz ES, Deos PH, Norris HJ. Metaplastic carcinomas of the breast. II. Spindle cell carcinoma. Hum Pathol 1989;20(8):732–40.
6. Foschini MP, Dina RE, Eusebi V. Sarcomatoid neoplasms of the breast: proposed definitions for biphasic and monophasic sarcomatoid mammary carcinomas. Semin Diagn Pathol 1993;10(2):128–36.
7. Davis WG, Hennessy B, Babiera G, et al. Metaplastic sarcomatoid carcinoma of the breast with absent or minimal overt invasive carcinomatous component: a misnomer. Am J Surg Pathol 2005;29(11):1456–63.
8. Carter MR, Hornick JL, Lester S, et al. Spindle cell (sarcomatoid) carcinoma of the breast: a clinicopathologic and immunohistochemical analysis of 29 cases. Am J Surg Pathol 2006;30(3):300–9.
9. Koker MM, Kleer CG. p63 expression in breast cancer: a highly sensitive and specific marker of metaplastic carcinoma. Am J Surg Pathol 2004;28(11):1506–12.
10. Leibl S, Gogg-Kammerer M, Sommersacher A, et al. Metaplastic breast carcinomas: are they of myoepithelial differentiation? immunohistochemical profile of the sarcomatoid subtype using novel myoepithelial markers. Am J Surg Pathol 2005;29(3):347–53.
11. Reis-Filho JS, Milanezi F, Steele D, et al. Metaplastic breast carcinomas are basal-like tumours. Histopathology 2006;49(1):10–21.
12. Gobbi H, Simpson JF, Borowsky A, et al. Metaplastic breast tumors with a dominant fibromatosis-like phenotype have a high risk of local recurrence. Cancer 1999;85(10):2170–82.
13. Sneige N, Yaziji H, Mandavilli SR, et al. Low-grade (fibromatosis-like) spindle cell carcinoma of the breast. Am J Surg Pathol 2001;25(8):1009–16.
14. Gobbi H, Simpson JF, Jensen RA, et al. Metaplastic spindle cell breast tumors arising within papillomas, complex sclerosing lesions, and nipple adenomas. Mod Pathol 2003;16(9):893–901.
15. Wargotz ES, Norris HJ, Austin RM, et al. Fibromatosis of the breast. A clinical and pathological study of 28 cases. Am J Surg Pathol 1987;11(1):38–45.
16. Rosen PP, Ernsberger D. Mammary fibromatosis. A benign spindle-cell tumor with significant risk for local recurrence. Cancer 1989;63(7):1363–9.
17. Abraham SC, Reynolds C, Lee JH, et al. Fibromatosis of the breast and mutations involving the APC/beta-catenin pathway. Hum Pathol 2002;33(1):39–46.
18. Wargotz ES, Weiss SW, Norris HJ. Myofibroblastoma of the breast. Sixteen cases of a distinctive benign mesenchymal tumor. Am J Surg Pathol 1987;11(7):493–502.
19. Hamele-Bena D, Cranor ML, Sciotto C, et al. Uncommon presentation of mammary myofibroblastoma. Mod Pathol 1996;9(7):786–90.
20. Nucci MR, Fletcher CDMF. Myofibroblastoma of the breast: a distinctive benign stromal tumor. Pathology Case Reviews 1999;4(5):214–9.

21. Magro G, Bisceglia M, Michal M, et al. Spindle cell lipoma-like tumor, solitary fibrous tumor and myofibroblastoma of the breast: a clinico-pathological analysis of 13 cases in favor of a unifying histogenetic concept. Virchows Arch 2002;440(3): 249–60.

22. Pauwels P, Sciot R, Croiset F, et al. Myofibroblastoma of the breast: genetic link with spindle cell lipoma. J Pathol 2000;191(3):282–5.

23. Weiss SW, Goldblum JR. Enzinger and Weiss's soft tissue tumors. 5th edition. Philadelphia: Mosby Elsevier; 2008.

LESIONS OF THE NIPPLE

Deborah A. Dillon, MD[a,b], Susan C. Lester, MD, PhD[a,b],*

KEYWORDS

- Nipple • Squamous metaplasia of lactiferous ducts • Duct ectasia • Nipple adenoma
- Papilloma • Syringomatous adenoma • Toker cells • Paget disease

ABSTRACT

Because of the singular anatomic structure of the nipple, some breast lesions only occur at this site. The overlying skin includes normal Toker cells near the duct orifices. These cells are occasionally so numerous as to be called Toker cell hyperplasia. Ductal carcinoma in situ (DCIS) may involve nipple skin by direct extension from the underlying ducts (Paget disease of the nipple). The numerous skin appendages (eg, sebaceous, apocrine, and eccrine glands[1]) in the nipple and areola are the likely origin of syringomatous adenomas. At the duct orifices, the normal squamous epithelium dips into the breast for a short distance and abruptly transitions to glandular luminal and myoepithelial cells. When keratin-producing cells extend deeper into the ducts, the condition of squamous metaplasia of lactiferous ducts (SMOLD) results. With age, the lactiferous sinuses are subject to weakened duct walls, inspissated secretions, and rupture, which result in the inflammatory masses or nipple discharge associated with duct ectasia. Superficial epithelial proliferations within the large lactiferous sinuses form nipple adenomas, and deeper proliferations often result in large-duct papillomas. Below the areola is a supporting smooth muscle layer that can give rise to leiomyomas, although these tumors are extraordinarily rare. The proximity of these lesions to the skin results in the majority of them presenting as palpable masses, skin changes, or nipple discharge. Biopsy specimens from these lesions may be small, superficial, or fragmented because of concern about maintaining the cosmetic appearance of the nipple and areola. Knowledge of the location of the biopsy, and the clinical presentation, is often essential in making the correct diagnosis.

SQUAMOUS METAPLASIA OF LACTIFEROUS DUCTS

OVERVIEW

This lesion goes by a variety of names: squamous metaplasia of lactiferous ducts (SMOLD), recurrent subareolar abscess, periductal mastitis, and Zuska disease.[2–10] The clinical presentation is of a painful, erythematous, subareolar mass. Typically, these findings are interpreted to be due to an acute bacterial infection, as is commonly seen in women during the lactational period. However, incision, drainage, and treatment using antibiotics directed toward *Staphylococci* rarely completely resolve the process (ergo, the name "recurrent subareolar abscess"). With recurrences, a fistula

Key Features
LESIONS OF THE NIPPLE

1. The majority of nipple lesions present with clinical symptoms or signs.

2. Many biopsy specimens are small, fragmented, or superficial because of concern about the cosmetic appearance of the nipple.

3. The clinical presentation is often helpful in arriving at the correct diagnosis, especially when the tissue available for evaluation is limited.

4. The majority of nipple lesions are benign. Overdiagnosis of malignancy exacts a high cost because many centrally located cancers will be treated by mastectomy.

[a] Harvard Medical School, 25 Shattuck Street, Boston, MA 02114 USA
[b] Department of Pathology, Brigham and Women's Hospital, 75 Francis Street, Boston, MA 02115, USA
* Corresponding author. Department of Pathology, Brigham and Women's Hospital, 75 Francis Street, Boston, MA 02115.
E-mail address: slester@partners.org (S.C. Lester).

Surgical Pathology 2 (2009) 391–412
doi:10.1016/j.path.2009.02.010

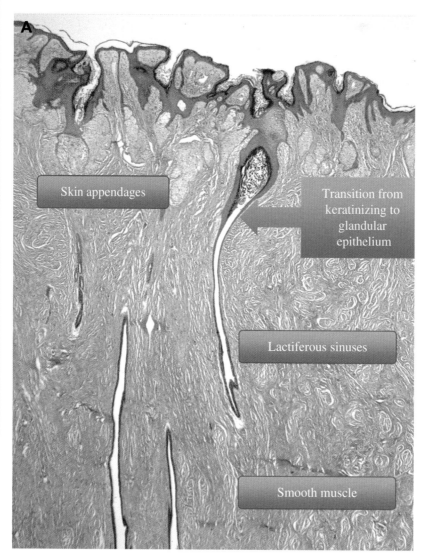

Fig. 1. (*A*) Normal nipple anatomy. The squamous surface epithelium dips into the nipple orifices. There is an abrupt transition to the glandular luminal and myoepithelial cells lining the lactiferous sinuses. Numerous accessory skin appendages are present in the nipple and areolar region. In the deep dermis, the nipple and areola are supported by a smooth muscle layer.

tract may burrow below the supporting smooth muscle of the nipple and erupt at the edge of the areola.

In the normal breast, the squamous cells of the skin dip into the duct orifice only a millimeter or two.[5] A keratin plug that forms in the orifice can be easily dislodged (**Fig. 1**A). If the squamous cells extend deeper into the duct, the keratin becomes trapped within the large duct system (**Fig. 1**B). When an involved duct ruptures, the keratin debris spills into the stroma and incites a foreign-body chronic active inflammatory response (**Fig. 2**A, B). Bacteria do not play a role in the primary lesion. However, with multiple surgical manipulations, bacterial superinfection may occur. The infections are often polymicrobial and anaerobic.

Women and men from a wide age range are affected, and almost all of those affected have a history of cigarette smoking.[11–13] It has been suggested that tobacco exposure could directly cause squamous metaplasia or that it could be a secondary effect of the decreased levels of beta carotene in smokers.[14]

GROSS APPEARANCE

Initial specimens are often from an incision and drainage procedure and generally consist of multiple small fragments of tissue without recognizable gross features. Skin usually is not present. If a definitive nipple wedge resection is performed, the specimen should be carefully oriented to distinguish skin from squamous metaplasia in ducts.

Fig. 1. (*B*) The keratinizing squamous cells extend deep into the nipple ducts, with keratin debris trapped within the lactiferous sinuses.

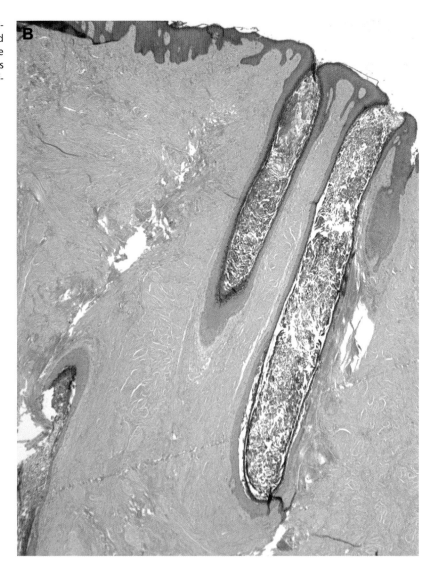

MICROSCOPIC FINDINGS

The diagnosis is often difficult to make using the typical fragmented specimen. There is usually a chronic active inflammatory infiltrate with scattered giant cells (**Fig. 2**A). If keratin debris is present within giant cells, this finding strongly supports the diagnosis. In poorly oriented specimens, it may be difficult to distinguish skin from keratinizing squamous metaplasia in large ducts.

In a definitive nipple resection, it may be possible to identify squamous metaplasia in deep ducts, ducts filled with keratin debris, and areas of rupture and spillage of keratin into the surrounding stroma (**Fig. 2**B). Well-formed granulomas would be an unusual finding. In general, only the nipple and subareolar tissue are involved.

DIFFERENTIAL DIAGNOSIS

The majority of patients will have had multiple surgical interventions before the diagnosis is made and a definitive surgical procedure is performed. Therefore, it is often difficult to distinguish the primary lesion with squamous metaplasia from changes due to prior surgery or subsequent bacterial infection. Often, diagnostic features of SMOLD are not present and the process is confused with that of duct ectasia or nonspecific postsurgical changes. Duct ectasia is not associated with squamous metaplasia when it is clearly distinguished from SMOLD.[11] Duct ectasia is predominantly a fibrotic reaction, with the inflammatory cells centered around multiple enlarged ducts. The chronic inflammatory reaction is caused by

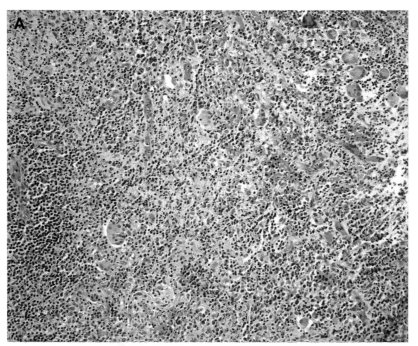

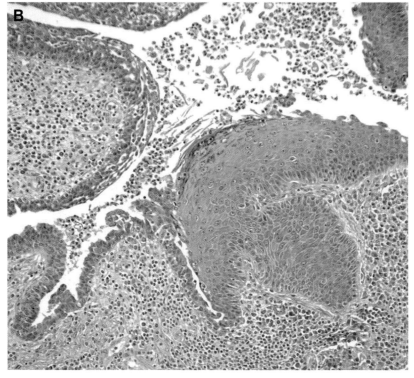

Fig. 2. (*A*) The typical incision-and-drainage specimen from patients who have SMOLD consists of a mixed inflammatory infiltrate with scattered giant cells and, in some cases, keratin debris. (*B*) Definitive excisions may demonstrate squamous metaplasia deep in the breast, entrapped keratin in ducts, and rupture into the adjacent stroma.

secretions, not keratin. Abscesses caused by bacterial infections associated with breastfeeding are typically deeper in the breast. A neutrophilic infiltrate will predominate, and cultures will be positive for *Staphylococci* or, less commonly, *Streptococci*.

The inflammatory infiltrate of SMOLD is sometimes described as granulomatous mastitis

Fig. 2. (*C*) The periductal fibrotic response in duct ectasia can closely mimic that of an irregular invasive carcinoma. (*D*) The surrounding chronic inflammation in this sample is the result of duct rupture and spillage of secretory material, not keratin, into the stroma.

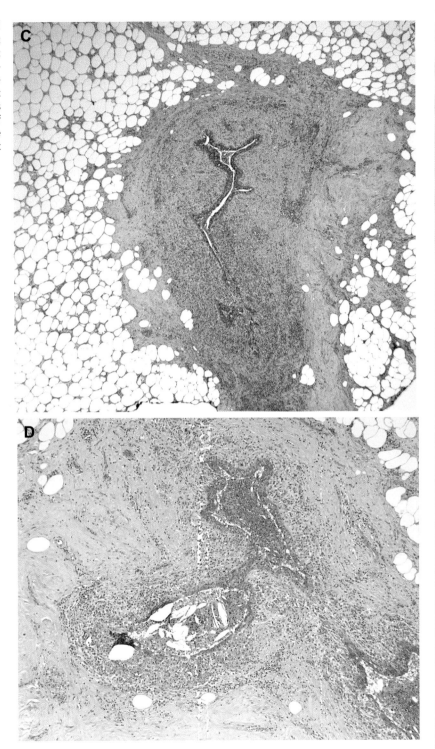

because of the presence of giant cells. This leads to confusion with the specific and different disease granulomatous lobular mastitis, which occurs deeper in the breast and is characterized by well-formed granulomas centered on ducts and lobules.[15–17] The presentation is usually as a painful, palpable mass, but the mass is generally not associated with the nipple.[18,19] Fistulas may form, but they are not typically periareolar. Affected individuals are almost all parous women. There is no association with smoking.[20] It is very important to distinguish SMOLD from granulomatous lobular mastitis because steroids are sometimes used to treat granulomatous lobular mastitis. This would be inappropriate treatment for SMOLD and could be detrimental if a secondary bacterial infection is present.

SMOLD can sometimes be mistaken for an epidermal inclusion cyst of the nipple or areola. The pathologic lesions are identical, except that SMOLD occurs within a duct orifice. Because of the cosmetic concerns at the nipple, the lesion is not fully excised as would occur at other sites, thus resulting in spillage of keratin into the stroma and the common history of multiple recurrences.

Squamous cells from the skin can be introduced into the breast during surgical procedures and the associated keratin debris can cause an inflammatory response. However, the location at the site of a prior surgical procedure away from the nipple will distinguish these cases from SMOLD.

DIAGNOSIS

The diagnosis of SMOLD often relies heavily on a clinical history of a painful erythematous subareolar mass in a nonlactating woman because the initial surgical procedure is rarely the definitive excision. In the appropriate clinical setting, in association with the finding of an abscess with a chronic inflammatory cellular infiltrate and scattered giant cells, the pathologist can suggest the diagnosis.

PROGNOSIS

If the duct in which SMOLD is present is not removed, recurrences are common.[14] The failure of treatment directed toward the incorrect clinical impression of a simple bacterial infection often leads to frustration on the part of the patient and physicians. Some patients have been accused of having Munchausen syndrome or have undergone subcutaneous mastectomy, a procedure that removes all breast tissue except the causative lesion. Unfortunately, the diagnosis often only becomes evident after multiple recurrences.

Appropriate treatment of SMOLD requires removal of the offending duct and excision of the fistula tract, if present. The number of recurrences after definitive surgery is greatly reduced.[14,21] Anecdotal evidence suggests that cessation of smoking can also reduce the likelihood of a recurrence.

DUCT ECTASIA

OVERVIEW

The occurrence of duct ectasia (also called plasma cell mastitis or comedomastitis) increases with age, and it is most common in older women. Lactiferous sinuses lose their supporting elastic fibers, and secretory material can accumulate. If the weakened walls rupture, the secretions are released into the stroma and incite a chronic inflammatory response. The periductal fibrosis can result in a palpable irregular mass that can closely mimic an invasive carcinoma and can cause skin retraction. Some patients may have a thick discharge from the nipple. This condition has not been associated with smoking.[11]

GROSS APPEARANCE

Due to the clinical presentation as a palpable mass or nipple discharge, excisional specimens generally remove the entire mass or resect the nipple duct region in continuity. Because many ducts are usually involved, the gross appearance is usually of an ill-defined, firm area.

MICROSCOPIC FINDINGS

In patients who have duct ectasia, large ectatic ducts are surrounded by a chronic inflammatory response (**Fig. 2**C). In lesions presenting as masses, associated periductal fibrosis is prominent around the ducts. There may be scattered giant cells, foamy histiocytes, lymphocytes, plasma cells, and pigment-laden macrophages in the surrounding stroma (**Fig. 2**D). However, well-formed granulomas are unusual. In older lesions, the lumen may be fibrotic with recanalization around the periphery, termed mastitis obliterans.

DIFFERENTIAL DIAGNOSIS

Periductal inflammation is also seen in SMOLD. However, in SMOLD, the inflammatory mass is the predominant feature. In duct ectasia, the inflammatory cells are generally confined to a region around the ducts and periductal fibrosis is the dominant feature. Squamous metaplasia is not a common feature of duct ectasia when it occurs separate from SMOLD.[11] Infectious diseases of the breast are exceedingly rare outside of the lactational period and are more commonly associated with either granulomas (eg, tuberculosis or fungal infections) or acute inflammation (eg, bacterial infections during lactation).

DIAGNOSIS

The diagnosis of duct ectasia is based on the histologic appearance as described under "Microscopic Features." In select cases, the use of special stains for organisms may be helpful to exclude the presence of an infectious process.

PROGNOSIS

Duct ectasia is a benign condition. Its only clinical importance is to distinguish the process from cancer. In many studies, this lesion is not well separated from those of SMOLD or those resulting from other inflammatory breast diseases.

NIPPLE ADENOMA

OVERVIEW

Various names have been used for this entity, including florid papillomatosis of the nipple, adenoma of the nipple, nipple duct adenoma, erosive adenomatosis, subareolar papillomatosis, and papillary adenoma of the nipple.[22-28] In part, the nomenclature reflects the broad range of histologic appearances that these lesions may display. The reported age range of patients with nipple adenoma is broad; however, the vast majority of adenomas occur in a person's fifth decade.

The lesion is similar in appearance to that of complex sclerosing lesions found deeper in the breast. However, because of their location in the superficial lactiferous ducts, clinical examination for nipple adenomas usually produces findings. Many form small palpable masses below the nipple skin. If the glandular epithelium grows onto the skin surface, or if there is trauma to the surface, the appearance may simulate erosion due to an invasive carcinoma (ie, erosive adenomatosis).[29,30] Other skin changes may be present, including erythema and crusting, which, when present, raise suspicion for Paget disease in the clinical differential diagnosis. In addition, some cases are associated with nipple discharge, which may be bloody. Imaging studies may show an irregular mass, raising the possibility of malignancy.

GROSS APPEARANCE

In the majority of cases, the lesion is small (less than 1 cm) and is not apparent during gross examination of the specimen.

MICROSCOPIC FEATURES

Nipple adenomas are relatively circumscribed because they arise within the large ducts of the nipple (Fig. 3A). Some may have an infiltrative appearance, particularly if they are sclerotic (Fig. 3D). The histologic appearance ranges from the proliferation of small ducts, similar to that seen in sclerosing adenosis, to the exuberant proliferation of papillary structures with associated epithelial hyperplasia, similar to that seen in benign papillary lesions elsewhere in the breast. Squamous epithelium may line some of the glandular spaces, or the cells may exhibit apocrine metaplasia. Mitoses and focal necrosis may be present and are not indicative of malignancy in the absence of overtly malignant cytology and architecture (Fig. 3C).

DIFFERENTIAL DIAGNOSIS

Nipple adenomas can show considerable intraductal proliferative activity, which, in some cases, may raise the possibility of in situ carcinoma. The presence of necrosis, in particular, may suggest the presence of DCIS (Fig. 3C). However, the cytologic features of the cellular proliferation will favor the diagnosis of a benign polyclonal proliferation. DCIS typically involving the nipple is of high nuclear grade and also involves the overlying nipple skin as Paget disease. However, Toker cell hyperplasia over a nipple adenoma can also raise the possibility of DCIS.[31]

Complex sclerosing adenosis associated with a nipple adenoma may need to be distinguished from invasive carcinoma. Immunoperoxidase studies can be used to document the presence of myoepithelial cells in adenomas (eg, p63, smooth muscle actin, or smooth muscle myosin heavy chain; Fig. 3D). Although there may be significant epithelial proliferation within the ducts, the myoepithelial cell layer is always retained in nipple adenomas. Invasive carcinoma may involve the nipple, but it does so either by direct extension from an invasive carcinoma present in the underlying breast tissue or as the recurrence of a previously excised invasive breast carcinoma. Adequate sampling and a complete clinical history are often helpful to exclude this possibility.

Syringomatous adenoma enters into the differential diagnosis process in lesions that have a predominantly glandular pattern and little intraductal proliferation. These lesions resemble syringomatous tumors arising at other sites. The clinical presentation of syringomatous adenoma in the nipple is similar to that of nipple adenoma; however, histologic distinction is usually possible based on the presence of

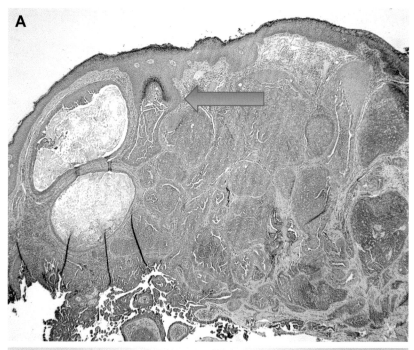

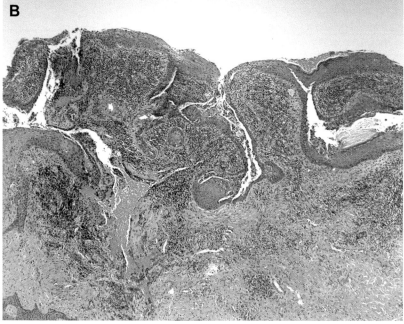

Fig. 3. (*A*) Nipple adenomas are present below the skin surface and consist of solid, papillary, and cystic areas. The involvement of a duct orifice can be seen (*arrow*). (*B*) Growth of glandular cells onto the surface, or trauma, can result in skin erosion or ulceration.

elongated, comma-shaped or branching ducts of the former. Myoepithelial cells may be difficult to identify using routine stains, but they can be detected using myoepithelial markers.

Squamous differentiation may be present, and keratotic cysts may also be seen.

Metaplastic spindle cell carcinomas or adenosquamous carcinomas can arise within nipple

Fig. 3. (*C*) Focal necrosis may be present in the center of nests of florid hyperplasia. (*D*) Results of an immunohistochemical study, performed because of concern for the presence of invasive carcinoma, show the presence of p63-positive myoepithelial cells in association with keratin-positive luminal cells (cytokeratin AE1/AE3, red = cytoplasm; p63, brown = nuclear).

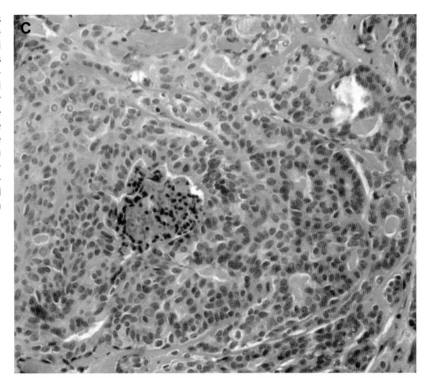

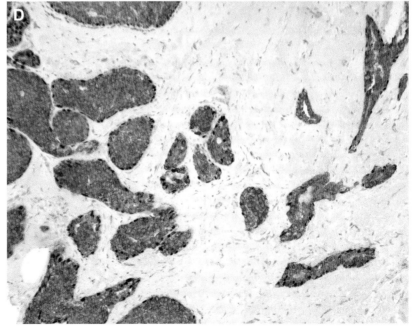

adenomas.[32] The diagnosis of carcinoma should be suspected when atypical spindle-shaped cells are present within the stroma. The malignant nature of the cells can be confirmed using immunohistochemical studies for broad spectrum and basal cytokeratins.

DIAGNOSIS

The diagnosis of nipple adenomas is generally based on the histologic appearance and the knowledge that the lesion is located at the nipple. Immunoperoxidase studies are occasionally necessary to exclude other diagnoses.

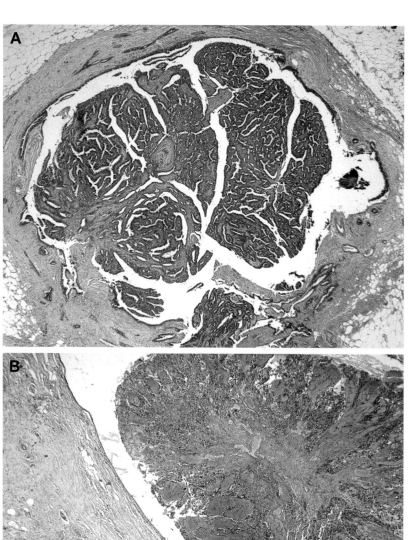

Fig. 4. (*A*) Large duct papillomas grow within lactiferous sinuses below the nipple. (*B*) The papillary fronds can twist and infarct, sometimes resulting in bloody nipple discharge.

PROGNOSIS

• Nipple adenomas should be completely excised, even when this requires excision of the nipple. Recurrence of incompletely excised lesions may occur.[33] In a small number of cases,[34] carcinoma has been reported to arise in association with an adenoma and, based on the presence of transitional areas, appears to arise, at least in some cases, within the adenoma.[35]

Fig. *4.* (*C*) Adjacent to a papilloma (to the left of the micrograph), epithelial nests are entrapped in the periductal fibrotic response (*arrow*). Immunoperoxidase studies are helpful to document the presence of p63-positive myoepithelial cells associated with keratin-positive luminal cells (brown = p63, nuclear; red = cytokeratin AE1/AE3, cytoplasm). (*D*) Isolated keratin-positive cells, some associated with myoepithelial cells (arrow), are sometimes identified in lymph nodes after a patient has had a core needle biopsy of a benign papillary lesion (immunohistochemical study as in Fig. 4C).

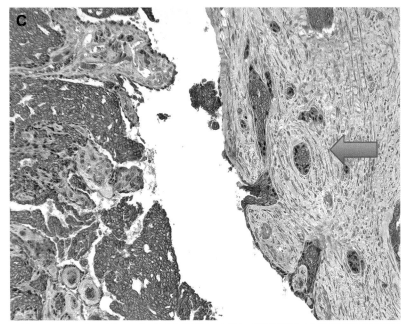

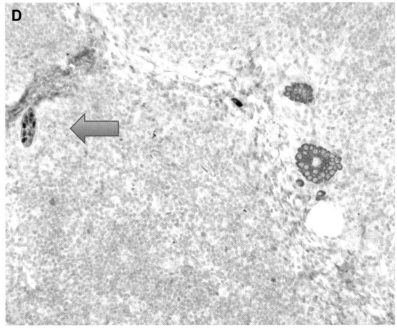

LARGE DUCT PAPILLOMA

OVERVIEW

Intraductal papillomas arising in the lactiferous sinuses are the most common nipple lesions.[36–38]

The majority of these lesions come to clinical attention because of their association with nipple discharge. The discharge can be bloody, if there has been infarction, and can be quite clinically alarming. Few are large enough to be palpable, but some can be visualized using ultrasound or mammography. The use of ductography generally reveals an intraductal filling defect, but this can be a difficult procedure to perform.

GROSS APPEARANCE

A nipple duct excision is generally performed to remove a known or suspected large duct papilloma. Because the papillary fronds are soft and pliable, they are generally difficult to palpate or see during gross examination. In rare instances, an outgrowth will be grossly apparent within a dilated duct.

MICROSCOPIC FINDINGS

The papilloma has a stalk and extends from the wall of a lactiferous sinus (**Fig. 4**A). The fibrovascular cores may be lined by a normal, two-cell layer, or florid epithelial hyperplasia may be present. Apocrine metaplasia is common and is a typical finding in benign papillomas.

DIFFERENTIAL DIAGNOSIS

Benign papillomas must be distinguished from papillary carcinomas.[36,37] Encapsulated (also termed intracystic) papillary carcinomas are usually deeper within the breast, but are also sometimes associated with nipple discharge (see separate article in this issue). Immunohistochemical studies will show evidence of myoepithelial cells within papillomas, and these cells will be absent in cases of papillary invasive carcinoma and DCIS. The muscle-type markers for myoepithelial cells (eg, smooth muscle actin, smooth muscle myosin heavy chain, and calponin) are also positive in the blood vessels that are often closely aligned along the base of the cells in the fibrovascular cores of papillary carcinomas. Therefore, antibodies to p63, which is not found in blood vessels, are generally a better marker for this purpose.

Epithelial nests can be entrapped within the surrounding fibrotic capsule.[39] The prior use of core needle biopsies can also push papillary fronds into the stroma.[36,37] These benign findings can usually be recognized as a result of their presence only within the inflamed stroma and by their association with myoepithelial cells (**Fig. 4**C). If a sentinel node biopsy is performed, small clusters of keratin positive cells are occasionally present (**Fig. 4**D). It has been suggested that benign cells can be transported to draining nodes as artifacts.[40] If the presence of myoepithelial cells can be demonstrated, the cells can be proven to be benign (**Fig. 4**D). If myoepithelial cells are absent, care must be taken not to overinterpret such cells as being indicative of metastatic carcinoma.

In rare cases, metaplastic spindle cell or adenosquamous carcinomas can arise within a papilloma.[32] The diagnosis of such conditions can be particularly difficult if there has been infarction of the papilloma associated with squamous metaplasia and an exuberant, reactive stromal response. Atypical-appearing spindle-shaped cells in the stroma may be identified as epithelial using immunohistochemical studies for cytokeratins. It may be necessary to use broad spectrum keratins that include basal-type keratins or specific antibodies for cytokeratins 14 and 17.

DIAGNOSIS

The diagnosis of large duct papilloma is based on the histologic appearance of the lesion and the presence of a myoepithelial cell layer. In selected cases, immunohistochemical studies can be of value.

PROGNOSIS

Papillomas are benign lesions. Removal is indicated to treat spontaneous nipple discharge and to exclude a diagnosis of carcinoma.

SYRINGOMATOUS ADENOMA

OVERVIEW

Syringomatous adenoma is a rare benign lesion, thought to arise from the eccrine glands of the nipple and areolar skin.[41,42] Most cases of syringomatous adenoma present as palpable subareolar masses. Some of the masses are painful and a few are associated with nipple discharge. There is a wide age range of patients with this condition, from prepubertal to elderly women. One case has been reported in a man.

GROSS APPEARANCE

The lesion is usually excised as a skin excision. An ill-defined, firm mass in the subcutaneous tissue may be discerned.

MICROSCOPIC FINDINGS

The lesion consists of small, well-formed nests of tumor cells in the dermis (**Fig. 5**A).[43] Many of the nests show squamous differentiation and are in the classic comma-shaped form. Glandular structures may be lined with eosinophilic material (**Fig. 5**B). A myoepithelial cell layer is evident using hematoxylin-eosin staining and can be confirmed using immunohistochemical studies. Mitotic

Fig. 5. (*A*) A syringoma-tous adenoma is composed of small nests of cells infiltrating in the dermis. In this image, the lesion infiltrates around a lactiferous sinus. (*B*) The tumor cell nests consist of clusters of squamous cells with typical comma-like shapes or glandular structures lined by dense eosinophilic material. A normal sebaceous gland is located to the right of the tumor.

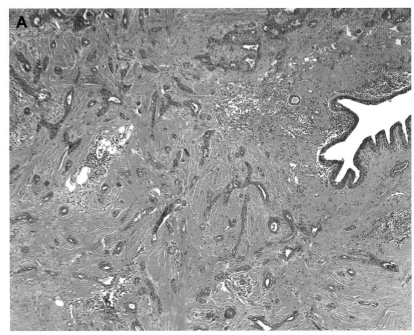

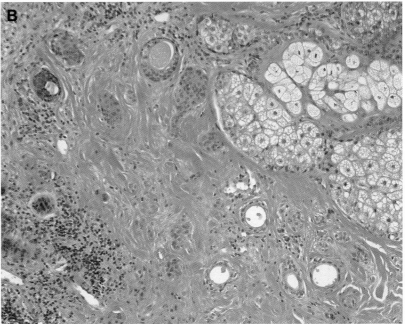

figures should be absent or rare. The lesion can infiltrate into the smooth muscle of the areola, and perineural invasion has been described. The cells should not penetrate into subcutaneous breast tissue or into the overlying skin.

DIFFERENTIAL DIAGNOSIS

The most important lesion to consider in the differential diagnosis of syringomatous adenoma is low-grade adenosquamous carcinoma. Whereas adenomas are restricted to the dermis, low-grade

A

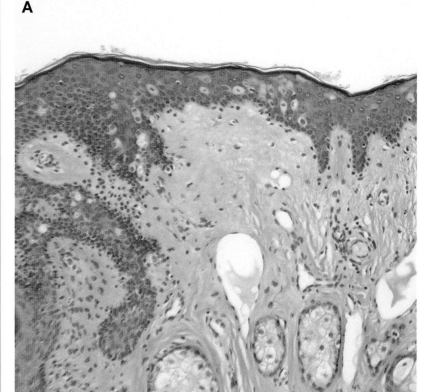

Fig. 6. (*A*) Toker cells are found in the nipple skin and cluster near nipple duct orifices.

adenosquamous carcinomas generally occur deeper in the breast. However, the histologic appearance of both lesions is similar, if not identical. There are rare reports of patients dying of breast cancer with metastases from low-grade adenosquamous carcinoma.[44] Therefore, a diagnosis stating that a tumor is benign should not be rendered unless the entire lesion is available for evaluation.

Syringomatous adenoma should never be mistaken for an invasive tubular carcinoma. A tubular carcinoma will lack myoepithelial cells and squamous differentiation, and will be present deeper in the breast. Tubular carcinomas are positive for estrogen receptor (ER) and progesterone receptor (PR); syringomatous adenomas are negative for these markers.

Nipple adenomas and syringomatous adenomas both may present clinically as subareolar masses. However, the microscopic appearances are distinct. Nipple adenomas are circumscribed or multilobated expansile hyperplasias within ducts, whereas syringomatous adenomas infiltrate as small nests of cells around normal structures.

DIAGNOSIS

The diagnosis of syringomatous adenoma is based on the histologic appearance of the lesion and on its location being restricted to nipple skin. If the specimen is only from a superficial biopsy, a deeper excision may be necessary to exclude the presence of a deeper carcinoma invading into the skin.

PROGNOSIS

Syringomatous adenomas are benign lesions. However, local recurrence has been reported, and complete excision is recommended.[42]

TOKER CELLS

OVERVIEW

Toker cells are normal components of the nipple skin and are most numerous around the nipple orifices. Toker cells were first well described by Dr. Cyril Toker, who recognized the possibility of these cells being mistaken for those in Paget disease.[45,46] The cells can be seen in about 10%

Fig. 6. (*B*) Toker cells have bland nuclei and abundant eosinophilic or clear cytoplasm. Occasional clusters or glands may be present.

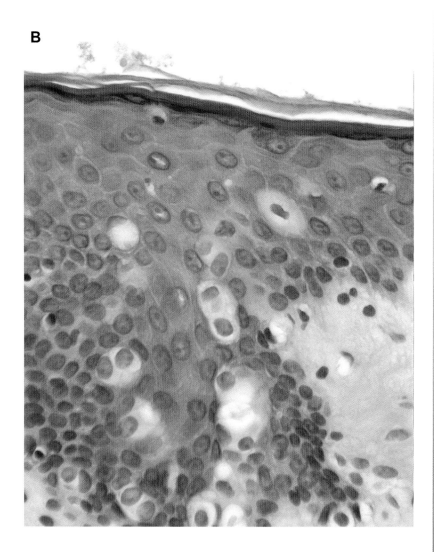

B

of nipples on routine stains. However, if immuno-histochemical studies are performed for cytokeratins found in luminal cells (eg, cytokeratin 7 or CAM5.2), Toker cells will be found in samples from up to 80% of nipples. In a few cases, the numbers of Toker cells are increased to a degree that the condition can be considered to be Toker cell hyperplasia.

GROSS APPEARANCE

Toker cells are found within normal nipple skin. There is no associated gross finding.

MICROSCOPIC FINDINGS

Toker cells have enlarged nuclei and clear cytoplasm and are located in the epidermis (**Fig. 6**A).

Rarely, the cells are clustered or form tubules. There should be minimal nuclear pleomorphism (**Fig. 6**B). The cells do not disrupt the tight junctions of the keratinocytes, and their presence does not result in the scale crust characteristic of Paget disease. The underlying lactiferous sinuses are normal in appearance. Toker cells have the appearance and immunoprofile characteristic of normal luminal cells—immunoreactive for cytokeratin 7 or CAM5.2, and estrogen or progesterone receptors (**Fig. 6**C; **Table 1**).[47] The cells are most numerous at the nipple duct orifices (**Fig. 6**D).[48]

DIFFERENTIAL DIAGNOSIS

Toker cells must be distinguished from those of DCIS. The cells of DCIS generally have marked

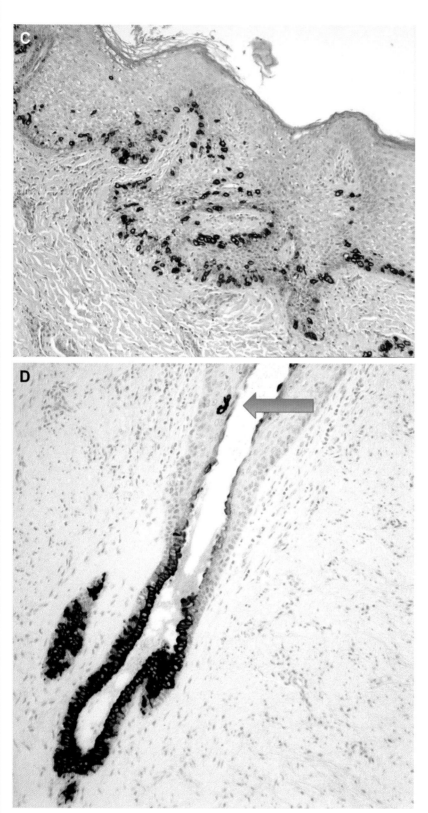

Fig. 6. (*C*) Toker cells are immunoreactive for cytokeratin 7 and CAM5.2 (brown = cytoplasm). (*D*) Luminal cells in a lactiferous sinus show positive results for cytokeratin 7 and CAM5.2. The more superficial squamous cells are not immunoreactive. A Toker cell is seen in the duct orifice (*arrow*).

nuclear pleomorphism and disrupt the tight junction of the keratinocytes. A scale crust is usually apparent and is usually the reason the patient comes to clinical attention. DCIS almost always involves the underlying ducts and lobules, although this may not be seen in a small biopsy or may be missed if the specimen is not oriented well.

Immunoperoxidase studies can be helpful. Toker cells have the same immunoprofile as normal luminal cells. In the majority of cases, DCIS involving nipple skin will be strongly HER2 positive (see **Table 1**).[47,49,50,51] Toker cells will not be positive for HER2. However, in some cases it may be difficult to interpret weak equivocal positivity. In such cases, the patient's clinical history, the location of the cells, and the lack of nuclear pleomorphism will help to exclude the diagnosis of DCIS.

There has been one reported case of lobular carcinoma in situ (LCIS) involving the nipple skin of a woman with bilateral LCIS deeper in the breast.[52] The cells in the skin were morphologically and immunohistochemically similar to Toker cells.[53] Although the cells in question were later reported to be negative for E-cadherin, supporting the classification as lobular neoplasia,[54] this marker has not been studied in Toker cells. This would be difficult to do in the majority of cases because most Toker cells are present as single cells surrounded by E-cadherin–positive squamous cells. Although Toker cells are very common, LCIS involving lactiferous sinuses is rare. The clinical significance of LCIS involving nipple skin in a woman who has LCIS elsewhere in the breast is unclear.

DIAGNOSIS

Toker cells can be incidental findings in a diagnostic biopsy performed for a different lesion.

Overdiagnosis of the presence of Toker cells as Paget disease must be avoided, particularly when the cells are primarily detected after the performance of immunoperoxidase studies for cytokeratin.

PROGNOSIS

Toker cells are normal constituents of nipple skin. Toker suggested in his original paper that the cells may be precursor cells for some cases of Paget disease.[45] That this might occur is supported by rare cases of patients with Paget disease without underlying carcinoma and rare patients with Toker cells having atypical features.[47,55]

DUCTAL CARCINOMA INVOLVING NIPPLE SKIN (PAGET DISEASE OF THE NIPPLE)

OVERVIEW

DCIS arising in the ducts and lobules of the breast can also involve the overlying skin. The tumor cells may extend up the lactiferous sinuses and onto the skin without passing through the contiguous basement membrane lining the ducts and skin (**Fig. 1**A). The tumor cells disrupt the tight junctions of the squamous cells, allowing extracellular fluid to exude onto the surface. This results in the clinical appearance of an eczematous crusting and weeping eruption on the involved nipple.

Sir James Paget made the first observation that women who had a unilateral scaling nipple crust were often later diagnosed as having breast carcinoma.[56] Currently, approximately 50% of patients presenting with Paget disease of the nipple will be found to have an area of invasive carcinoma deeper in the breast. This is a rare presentation of breast cancer, only occurring in 1% to 4% of patients. Subclinical Paget disease can be found

---

Table 1
Immunohistochemical markers for epidermal lesions of nipple skin

	Cam 5.2 or CK7	S100	HMB45	GCDFP-15	HER2	ER/PR	E-cadherin	Mucin
Paget disease of the nipple	Positive	Low	Negative	Moderate	High	Low	High	High
Squamous cell carcinoma	Low	Low	Negative	Negative	Low	Negative	Positive	Negative
Melanoma	Low	Positive	Positive	Negative	Negative	Negative	Negative	Negative
Toker cells	Positive	Negative	Negative	Low	Negative	High	Unknown	Negative
LCIS	Positive	Negative	Negative	Moderate	Negative	Positive	Negative	High

Abbreviation: LCIS, lobular carcinoma in situ.
Key: Positive, > 90% of cases; High, 60 to 90%; Moderate, 40 to 60%; Low, 10 to 30%; Negative, < 10%.

A

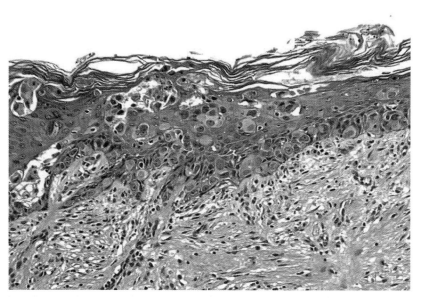

B

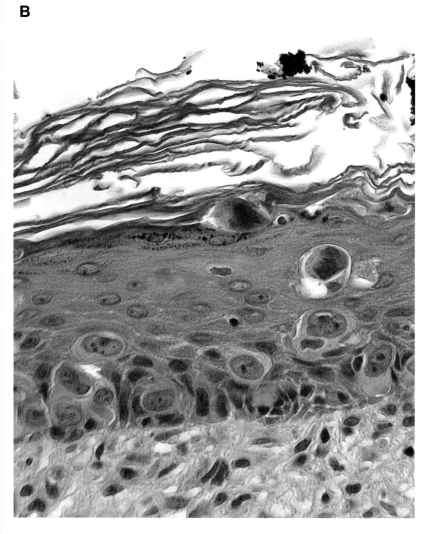

Fig. 7. (*A*) Paget disease is characterized by the presence of malignant cells, singly and in nests in nipple skin. The tight junctions of the squamous cells are disrupted, resulting in a scale crust. (*B*) The cells have enlarged hyperchromatic nuclei with prominent nucleoli.

Fig. 7. (*C*) Most cases of Paget disease will be strongly positive for HER2/neu (brown = membrane). (*D*) In rare cases, invasion can occur through the basement membrane of the skin. The invasive cells are positive for keratin (AE1/AE3, red = cytoplasm) and lack myoepithelial cells (p63, brown = nucleus).

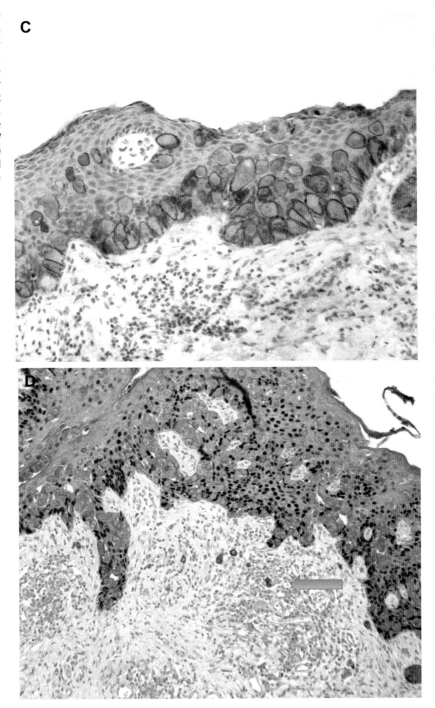

in a larger number of patients who undergo mastectomy for cancer.

Pagetoid spread is used as a general term for neoplastic cells that are present between a basement membrane and an overlying, intact normal epithelial layer. This pattern can also be seen at other sites, such as the vulva and anus. Within the ducts and lobules of the breast, pagetoid spread is almost always associated with atypical lobular hyperplasia and LCIS. It is less often seen in association with DCIS because DCIS generally grows as solid masses without preservation of preexisting normal luminal cells. However, in the skin, the overlying squamous cells are disrupted but not completely replaced by the Paget cells of DCIS.

GROSS APPEARANCE

The scale crust is generally cleaned off the nipple before a biopsy is performed. Therefore, a grossly evident lesion is usually not present in small diagnostic biopsy specimens. A prior skin punch biopsy site should not be mistaken for skin ulceration.

MICROSCOPIC FINDINGS

Single tumor cells and clusters of cells disrupt the tight junctions of keratinocytes, resulting in exudation of intracellular fluid and a scale crust (**Fig. 7**A). Scrapings of the scale crust can be used to make a cytologic diagnosis of Paget disease. The cells have large pleomorphic nuclei with prominent nucleoli and abundant amphophilic cytoplasm (**Fig. 7**B). The cells rarely form glandular structures.[57–59] The tumor cells in almost all cases are positive for HER2/neu (**Fig. 7**C).[50,51,60]

DCIS almost always involves the underlying ductal system. In rare cases, DCIS is restricted to the skin, without involvement of deeper breast tissue. In very rare cases, there is invasion through the basement membrane of the skin into the dermis (**Fig. 7**D).

DIFFERENTIAL DIAGNOSIS

Other malignancies of the skin to be considered include squamous cell carcinoma and melanoma.[60,61] However, these diagnoses are much rarer than that of Paget disease at this site. Only DCIS will also involve the underlying ducts. Immunoperoxidase studies can be helpful in making the diagnosis (see **Table 1**). DCIS will be positive for cytokeratin 7 and CAM5.2, whereas squamous cell carcinoma and melanoma will be negative for these markers.[60] Additional melanoma-specific markers can be used to support a diagnosis of melanoma. It should be noted that melanin can sometimes be found in Paget cells.

DIAGNOSIS

The diagnosis of Paget disease of the nipple is generally made because of the presence of diagnostic features of DCIS in the deeper portions of the breast, with similar-appearing cells in nipple skin. Immunohistochemical studies are sometimes helpful with small diagnostic biopsies.

Pitfalls
DIAGNOSIS OF LESIONS OF THE NIPPLE

1. The failure of clinicians and pathologists to recognize the pathogenesis of SMOLD often leads to inappropriate treatment, recurrence, and increased morbidity for patients.

2. Nipple adenomas and large duct papillomas may be mistaken for DCIS, intracystic papillary carcinoma, or invasive carcinoma when there is florid epithelial hyperplasia, focal necrosis, or a peripheral sclerosing pattern. Immunohistochemical studies can be helpful to demonstrate the presence of a well-formed myoepithelial layer.

3. Core needle biopsies of benign papillary lesions may push epithelial cells into the adjacent stroma or into lymphatics and lymph nodes. Immunohistochemical studies for the presence of myoepithelial cells and the recognition of the phenomenon will help prevent overdiagnosis of invasive carcinoma and metastatic disease.

4. Syringomatous adenomas may be overdiagnosed as invasive carcinomas because of their infiltrative pattern in the dermis. Determination of the location and extent of these lesions is essential to distinguish them from low-grade adenosquamous carcinomas that occur deeper in the breast.

5. Toker cells are normally present in nipple skin and are clinically occult. When they are numerous, they may be mistaken for Paget disease. The lack of clinical symptoms, the bland histologic appearance, the absence of involvement deeper in the breast, and the absence of HER2/neu expression will correctly identify most cases.

PROGNOSIS

The prognosis for Paget disease depends on the stage of the underlying carcinoma. Paget disease without invasive carcinoma is classified as DCIS (stage 0) and has an excellent prognosis.

REFERENCES

1. Giacometti L, Montagna W. The nipple and areola of the human female breast. Anat Rec 1962;144:191–7.
2. Zuska J, Crile G, Ayres W. Fistulas of lactiferous ducts. Am J Surg 1952;81:312–7.
3. Atkins HJB. Mamillary fistula. Br Med J 1955;2: 1473–4.
4. Patey DH, Thackray AC. Pathology and treatment of mammary-duct fistula. Lancet 1958;2:871–3.

5. Toker C. Lactiferous duct fistula. J Pathol Bacteriol 1962;84:143–6.

6. Habif D, Perzin K, Lipton R, et al. Subareolar abscess associated with squamous metaplasia of lactiferous ducts. Am J Surg 1970;119:423–6.

7. Crile G Jr, Chatty EM. Squamous metaplasia of lactiferous ducts. Arch Surg 1971;102:533–4.

8. Powell BC, Maull KI, Sachatello CR. Recurrent subareolar abscess of the breast and squamous metaplasia of the lactiferous ducts: a clinical syndrome. South Med J 1977;70:935–7.

9. Haagensen CD. Infections in the breast. Diseases of the breast. 3rd edition. Philadelphia: WB Saunders; 1986. p. 386–8.

10. Lester S. Subareolar abscess (Zuska's disease): a specific disease entity with specific treatment and prevention strategies. Pathology Case Reviews 1999;4:189–93.

11. Dixon JM, Ravisekar O, Chetty U, et al. Periductal mastitis and duct ectasia: different conditions with different aetiologies. Br J Surg 1996;82:820–2.

12. Schafer P, Furrer C, Mermillod B. An association of cigarette smoking with recurrent subareolar breast abscess. Int J Epidemiol 1988;17:810–3.

13. Bundred NJ, Dover MS, Coley S, et al. Breast abscesses and cigarette smoking. Br J Surg 1992;79:58–9.

14. Meguid M, Oler A, Numann PJ, et al. Pathogenesis-based treatment of recurring subareolar breast abscesses. Surgery 1995;118:775–82.

15. Going JJ, Anderson TJ, Wilkinson S, et al. Granulomatous lobular mastitis. J Clin Pathol 1987;40:535–40.

16. Kessler E, Wolloch Y. Granulomatous mastitis: a lesion clinically simulating carcinoma. Am J Clin Pathol 1972;58:642–6.

17. Cohen C. Granulomatous mastitis. A review of 5 cases. S Afr Med J 1977;52:14–6.

18. Baslaim M, Khayat HA, Al-Amoudi SA. Idiopathic granulomatous mastitis: a heterogeneous disease with variable clinical presentation. World J Surg 2007;31:1677–81.

19. Bani-Hani KE, Yaghan RJ, Matalka II, et al. Idiopathic granulomatous mastitis: time to avoid unnecessary mastectomies. Breast J 2004;10:318–22.

20. Al-Khaffaf B, Knox F, Bundred NJ. Idiopathic granulomatous mastitis: a 25-year experience. J Am Coll Surg 2008;206:269–73.

21. Li S, Grant CS, Degnim A, et al. Surgical management of recurrent subareolar breast abscesses: Mayo Clinic experience. Am J Surg 2006;192:528–9.

22. Diaz NM, Palmer JO, Wick MR. Erosive adenomatosis of the nipple: histology, immunohistology, and differential diagnosis. Mod Pathol 1992;5:179–84.

23. Oria C-M, LeGal Y, Dader P. L'adenomatose erosive de mamelon. Ann Anat Pathol 1959;4:292–304.

24. Handley RS, Thackray AC. Adenoma of the nipple. Br J Cancer 1962;16:187–94.

25. Jones DB. Florid papillomatosis of the nipple ducts. Cancer 1955;8:315–9.

26. Perzin KH, Lattes R. Papillary adenoma of the nipple (florid papillomatosis adenoma, adenomatosis). A clinicopathologic study. Cancer 1972;29:996–1009.

27. Shapiro L, Karpas CM. Florid papillomatosis of the nipple. First reported case in a male. Am J Clin Pathol 1965;44:155–9.

28. Nichols FC, Dockerty MB, Judd JE. Florid papillomatosis of the nipple. Surg Gynecol Obstet 1958;107:474–80.

29. Smith EJ, Kron SD, Gross PR. Erosive adenomatosis of the nipple. Arch Dermatol 1970;102:330–2.

30. Smith NP, Jones EW. Erosive adenomatosis of the nipple. Clin Exp Dermatol 1977;2:79–84.

31. Manavi M, Hudelist G, Schatten C, et al. Characteristics of clear cells and Toker cells in the epidermis of underlying nipple duct adenoma. Anticancer Res 2002;22:3691–700.

32. Gobbi H, Simpson JF, Jensen RA, et al. Metaplastic spindle cell breast tumors arising within papillomas, complex sclerosing lesions, and nipple adenomas. Mod Pathol 2003;16:893–901.

33. Taylor HB, Robertson AG. Adenoma of the nipple. Cancer 1965;18:995–1002.

34. Jones MW, Tavassoli FA. Coexistence of nipple duct adenoma and breast carcinoma: a clinicopathologic study of five cases and review of the literature. Mod Pathol 1995;8:633–6.

35. Rosen PP, Caicco JA. Florid papillomatosis of the nipple. A study of 51 patients, including nine with mammary carcinoma. Am J Surg Pathol 1986;10:87–101.

36. Collins LC, Schnitt SJ. Papillary lesions of the breast: selected diagnostic and management issues. Histopathology 2008;52:20–9.

37. Mulligan AM, O'Malley FP. Papillary lesions of the breast: a review. Anat Pathol 2007;14:108–19.

38. Haagensen CD, Stout AP, Phillips JS. The papillary neoplasms of the breast. I. Benign intraductal papilloma. Ann Surg 1951;133:18–36.

39. Nagi C, Bleiweiss I, Jaffer S. Epithelial displacement in breast lesions: a papillary phenomenon. Arch Pathol Lab Med 2005;129:1465–9.

40. Diaz NM, Vrcel V, Centeno BA, et al. Modes of benign mechanical transport of breast epithelial cells to axillary lymph nodes. Adv Anat Pathol 2005;12:7–9.

41. Carter E, Dyess DL. Infiltrating syringomatous adenoma of the nipple: a case report and 20-year retrospective review. Breast J 2004;10:443–7.

42. Ku J, Bennett RD, Chong KD, et al. Syringomatous adenoma of the nipple. Breast 2004;13:412–5.

43. Rosen PP. Syringomatous adenoma of the nipple. Am J Surg Pathol 1983;7:739–45.

44. Van Hoeven KH, Drudis T, Cranor ML, et al. Low-grade adenosquamous carcinoma of the breast. A clinicopathologic study of 32 cases with ultrastructural analysis. Am J Surg Pathol 1993;17:248–58.

45. Toker C. Clear cells of the nipple epidermis. Cancer 1970;25:601–10.

46. Martin-Reay D. What are Toker cells and who is Toker? Dermatopathology: practical and conceptual. Available at: http://www.derm101.com. Accessed April 1, 2009.

47. Di Tommaso L, Franchi G, Destro A, et al. Toker cells of the breast. Morphological and immunohistochemical characterization of 40 cases. Hum Pathol 2008; 39:1295–300.

48. Yao DX, Hoda SA, Chiu A, et al. Intraepidermal cytokeratin 7 immunoreactive cells in the non-neoplastic nipple may represent interepithelial extension of lactiferous duct cells. Histopathology 2002;40:230–6.

49. de Potter CR, Eeckout I, Schelfhout AM, et al. Keratinocyte induced chemotaxis in the pathogenesis of Paget's disease of the breast. Histopathology 1994; 24:349–56.

50. Anderson JM, Ariga R, Govil H, et al. Assessment of Her-2/Neu status by immunohistochemistry and fluorescence in situ hybridization in mammary Paget disease and underlying carcinoma. Appl Immunohistochem Mol Morphol 2003;11:120–4.

51. Bianco MK, Vasef MA. HER-2 gene amplification in Paget disease of the nipple and extramammary site: a chromogenic in situ hybridization study. Diagn Mol Pathol 2006;15:131–5.

52. Sahoo S, Green I, Rosen PP. Bilateral Paget disease of the nipple associated with lobular carcinoma in situ. Arch Pathol Lab Med 2002;126:90–2.

53. Fair KP. Bilateral Paget disease of the nipple. [letter to the editor]. Arch Pathol Lab Med 2002; 126:1159.

54. Rosen PP. Bilateral Paget disease of the nipple. [reply to letter to the editor]. Arch Pathol Lab Med 2002;126:1159.

55. Marucci G, Betts CM, Golouh R, et al. Toker cells are probably precursors of Paget cell carcinoma: a morphological and ultrastructural description. Virchows Arch 2002;441:117–23.

56. Paget J. On disease of the mammary areola preceeding cancer of the mammary gland. St. Bartholomew's Hospital Reports 1874;10:87–9.

57. Toker C. Some observations on Paget's disease of the nipple. Cancer 1961;14:653–71.

58. Shousha S. Glandular Paget's disease of the nipple. Histopathology 2007;50:812–4.

59. Toker C. Glandular Paget's disease of the nipple. [letter]. Histopathology 2008;52:767–83.

60. Lloyd J, Flanagan AM. Mammary and extramammary Paget's disease. J Clin Pathol 2000;53:742–9.

61. Kohler S, Rouse RV, Smoller BR. The differential diagnosis of pagetoid cells in the epidermis. Mod Pathol 1998;11:79–92.

MUCINOUS LESIONS OF THE BREAST

Jeong Yun Shim, MD, Aysegul A. Sahin, MD*

KEYWORDS

• Breast • Carcinoma • Lesion • Mammography • Mucin

ABSTRACT

Breast lesions associated with extracellular mucin production are uncommon and constitute a wide spectrum of lesions ranging from benign cyst to mucinous carcinoma. Intracytoplasmic mucin can be seen rarely in benign metaplasias but is a common finding in invasive and in situ carcinomas. In this article, we discuss the differential diagnosis of breast lesions associated with mucin production and other entities that show histologic changes that mimic mucin production.

Mucins are a family of high-molecular-weight glycoproteins produced by epithelial cells and are involved in diverse functions.[1] There are two structurally and functionally distinct classes of mucins: secreted gel-forming mucins and transmembrane mucins. At least 19 human mucin genes have been distinguished by cDNA cloning.[2,3] In normal breast epithelium, mucin expression is highly polarized to the apical surface. Loss of polarized expression of mucin by incomplete glycosylation, abnormal distribution, or ectopic expression is a characteristic of neoplastic transformation in breast epithelium.[4–6] Excessive mucin may be secreted indiscriminately into the tissue spaces (extracellular mucin) or retained as a large droplet in cytoplasm (intracellular mucin). Breast lesions associated with extracellular mucin production are uncommon and constitute a wide spectrum of lesions ranging from benign cyst to mucinous carcinoma. Intracytoplasmic mucin can be seen rarely in benign metaplasias but is a common finding in invasive and in situ carcinomas.[7–13]

In this article, we discuss the differential diagnosis of breast lesions associated with mucin production and other entities that show histologic changes that mimic mucin production.

BREAST LESIONS ASSOCIATED WITH EXTRACELLULAR MUCIN PRODUCTION

The spectrum of breast lesions that demonstrate extracellular mucin includes cyst, mucocele-like lesion, mucinous carcinoma, mucinous cystadenocarcinoma, and metastatic carcinoma.[8,12,13]

CYST

Microscopic breast cysts are common incidental findings that are considered aberrations of lobular involution. They occur most often as part of a spectrum of proliferative abnormalities referred to as fibrocystic changes. Most breast cysts contain granular eosinophilic secretory material; less commonly, mucus secretion can occur.

Gross Features

The majority of these lesions are incidental findings, and there is no specific gross pathology.

Microscopic Features

These lesions are lined by a single layer of either columnar epithelium or attenuated flattened cells (**Figs. 1** and **2**). Sometimes they have no identifiable epithelial lining at all. In general these cysts are incidental findings and measure less than a few millimeters. Microcalcifications can be found in the mucin-filled cysts.

Differential Diagnosis

Differential diagnosis includes mucocele-like lesion and cystic neoplastic lesions such as cystic

Department of Pathology, The University of Texas M. D. Anderson Cancer Center, Unit 085, Houston, TX 77030-4009, USA
* Corresponding author.
E-mail address: asahin@mdanderson.org (A.A. Sahin).

Surgical Pathology 2 (2009) 413–440
doi:10.1016/j.path.2009.02.011

hypersecretory carcinoma and adenoid cystic carcinoma. Cysts may rupture and mucin content may spill into stroma. Ruptured cysts associated with extracellular mucin can be distinguished from hypocellular mucinous carcinoma by the lack of epithelial cells in the mucus. Usually adjacent ducts also show different stages of cyst formation with distention. The lack of epithelial proliferation excludes other neoplastic processes (**Table 1**).

MUCOCELE-LIKE LESION

Mucocele-like lesion of the breast was first described in 1986 as a benign lesion composed of cystic spaces containing mucin with frequent rupture of the cyst wall and extravasation of secretions into the surrounding stroma analogous to mucocele of the minor salivary gland.[14] Subsequent reports have suggested that this lesion may be associated with epithelial proliferations such as hyperplasia without atypia and atypical ductal hyperplasia, papilloma, and both in situ and invasive cancer.[15–18] Because the main characteristic of this entity is the presence of abundant mucin with extravasation into stroma, it is better to define it as a lesion rather than a tumor and to classify the accompanying lesion as either a nonneoplastic epithelial proliferation or a benign or malignant neoplastic proliferation.

Gross Features

Mucocele-like lesions have been reported to present as a palpable mass, an asymptomatic

Key Features
MUCOCELE-LIKE LESION

1. Extravasation of mucin into the surrounding stroma

2. Cystically dilated and partially ruptured spaces containing mucin

3. Epithelial lining may be flat, attenuated, cuboidal, or papillary

4. Proliferative changes may occur in the lining epithelium

5. Histiocytes and inflammatory cells present in secretion but no detached epithelium

6. No fibrovascular septa in mucin pools

7. Coarse microcalcifications common

8. Clinical outcome is based on the nature of the lesion that accompanies mucocele-like lesion

mammographic abnormality, or an incidental finding.[16–20] On mammography, they may present either as an ill-defined mass with or without calcifications or as clustered, coarse calcifications.[19,20] Ultrasonographic findings include clustered, hypoechogenic, round or lobulated, solid or cystic lesions with or without echogenic spots. An increased number of microscopic mucocele-like

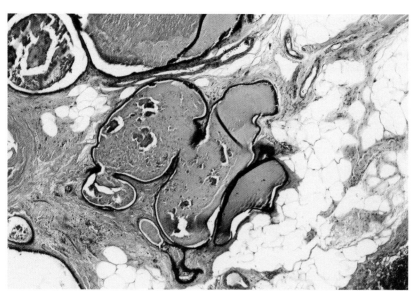

Fig. 1. **Benign cyst**. A cluster of dilated cysts with mucinous content, sometimes termed "unfolded lobules." This is a common finding on stereotactic core needle biopsies performed for microcalcifications.

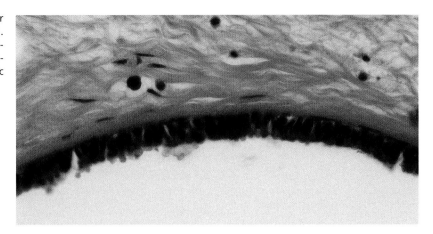

Fig. 2. **Benign cyst**. Higher magnification of **Fig. 1**. The wall is lined by flattened secretory epithelium without cytologic atypia.

lesions are identified on core needle biopsies among mammographically screened patients.[20]

The gross appearance may vary from the presence of only one or two small cystic spaces to an ill-defined mass-like lesion consisting of many cystic spaces containing mucinous material.

Microscopic Features

Many cystic spaces containing mucin with associated rupture and extravasation of mucin into the surrounding stroma are present (**Figs. 3–5**). The variable-sized cystic spaces are lined by flattened or cuboidal epithelium (**Fig. 6**). Attenuation or detachment of the lining epithelium is common (see **Fig. 4**). Columnar cell change or hyperplasia with or without atypia may be present.[18] Variable degrees of epithelial proliferative changes resembling usual ductal epithelial hyperplasia may also be seen in the cystic spaces (**Figs. 7** and **8**).[15–18] The mucin in mucocele-like lesions is usually neutral or contains nonsulfated acid, and can be positively stained by a periodic acid–Schiff, mucicarmine, or Alcian blue.[12]

Differential Diagnosis

Fibrocystic changes with mucin-filled cysts may resemble mucocele-like lesion on low magnification. However, rupture with extravasated mucin is not present in fibrocystic change. Myxoid degeneration of stroma encountered after a biopsy or chemotherapy is relatively common and may at times be difficult to differentiate from mucocele-like lesion. In this case, sections should be carefully evaluated for the presence of epithelial cells to rule out mucocele-like lesion. Other histologic changes associated with previous biopsy including scar-like stromal fibrosis, granulation tissue, hemorrhage and inflammation, and changes associated with previous chemotherapy such as stromal fibrosis, histiocytic infiltration, and increased vascularity should also be helpful in determining the differential diagnosis. Several other neoplasms including fibroadenoma or phyllodes tumor with myxoid change, mucinosis, and myxoma may partly resemble mucocele-like tumor. Myxoid stromal change is a common finding in fibroadenoma and phyllodes tumor.[21] However, mucin-filled cysts with rupture and extravasation of mucin

Table 1		
Differential diagnosis of mucinous lesions of the breast		
Extracellular Mucin	**Intracellular Mucin**	**Both Intracellular and Extracellular Mucin**
Mucinous cysts	Signet ring cell carcinoma	Secretory carcinoma
Mucocele-like lesion	Mucoepidermoid carcinoma	Adenoid cystic carcinoma
Mucinous carcinoma	Metastatic carcinoma	Metastatic carcinoma
Metastatic carcinoma		

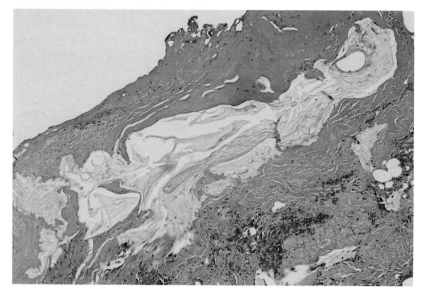

Fig. 3. Mucocele-like lesion. Acellular mucin is dissecting into stroma. No epithelial cells are seen adjacent to or within the dissecting mucin.

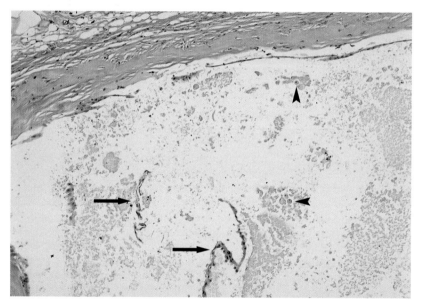

Fig. 4. Mucocele-like lesion. Detached strips of epithelium are present in the mucin (*arrows*) which should not be confused with mucinous carcinoma. Scattered macrophages are identified in mucin (*arrowheads*).

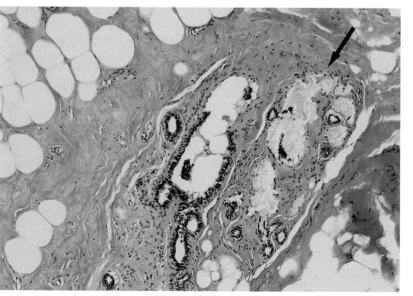

Fig. 5. Mucocele-like lesion. Focal spillage of mucin (*arrow*) was identified as an incidental microscopic finding on a mastectomy performed for invasive high-grade ductal carcinoma; this lesion was observed in a representative section of breast parenchyma away from tumor.

Fig. 6. Mucocele-like lesion. Cystically dilated and partially ruptured cysts lined by a proliferative epithelium and extravasation of mucin (arrow) into the breast parenchyma.

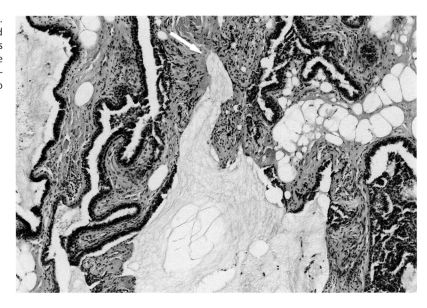

are not a feature of these entities. Mucinosis is another rare lesion composed of myxoid material.[22] Myxoma is a rare tumor consisting of hypocellular myxoid tissue containing spindle cells;[23] the absence of epithelial cells differentiates myxoma and mucinosis from mucocele-like lesion. It may be especially difficult to differentiate the above entities from mucocele-like lesion when mucin is present in the core biopsy. Because core biopsy material may contain limited tissue and the findings may be underdiagnosed or overdiagnosed, it is prudent to excise the entire lesion when mucin is present on core biopsy.[24,25] A paucicellular mucinous carcinoma with only a few tumor cells within a large extracellular mucin pool may make differentiation from mucocele-like lesions difficult, especially in a core biopsy specimen. In this case, multiple deeper sections

Fig. 7. Mucocele-like lesion. Higher magnification of Fig. 6. The epithelial lining shows usual hyperplasia.

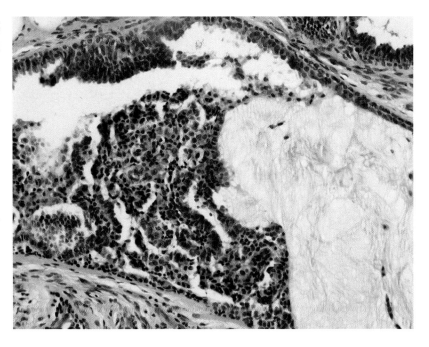

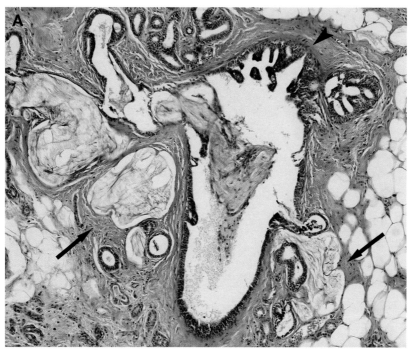

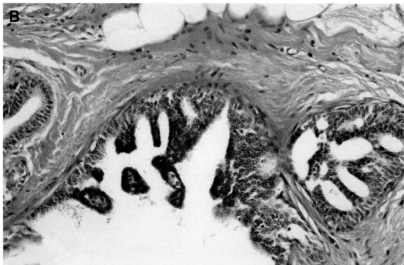

Fig. 8. (*A*) **Mucocele-like lesion** with atypical ductal hyperplasia. Most of the cystically dilated duct is lined by flat epithelium. The upper portion of the duct (*arrowheads*) has micropapillary architecture. Spillage of mucin is evident in multiple areas (*arrows*). (*B*) Higher magnification of upper portion of the cyst wall shows complex epithelial proliferation with micropapillary and cribriform architecture.

should be examined to determine whether epithelial cells are present. When epithelial cells are present, the absence of intact myoepithelial cells and of residual intact ductal epithelial lining favors the diagnosis of mucinous carcinoma over mucocele-like lesion. Rarely, epithelial cells are detached into the mucin-filled cyst or into the dissecting stromal mucin pool in mucocele-like lesion; in this situation the same criteria may be used to differentiate between the two entities. Immunohistochemical staining for myoepithelial cells may be helpful.

Prognosis

Although originally described as a benign lesion, mucocele-like lesions can be associated with other lesions, including hyperplasias and in situ and invasive malignancies. Therefore, we do not consider a mucocele-like lesion as a specific entity, but rather view it as histologic finding; the key to determining its prognosis is not the presence of the mucocele-like lesion itself, but rather the type of the lesion associated with the mucocele-like lesion.

MUCINOUS CARCINOMA

Mucinous carcinoma, also known as mucoid, gelatinous, or colloid carcinoma, is a rare type of invasive carcinoma, comprising about 2%–6% of all primary breast carcinomas.[26–31] As in other special types of breast cancers, mucinous carcinoma can be pure or mixed with other types of invasive breast cancers.[32] Mucinous carcinomas occur more commonly in postmenopausal women. The median age of patients who have pure mucinous carcinomas is over 65 years, which is older than patients who have conventional invasive ductal carcinomas.[12,13] Multicentricity or bilaterality is not a common finding. Mucinous carcinomas characteristically form a well-circumscribed mass lesion, and patients usually present with a palpable mass.[26–30]

Imaging Features

On mammography, pure mucinous carcinoma presents as a circumscribed, lobulated mass (**Figs. 9 and 10**).[33,34] Mixed mucinous carcinoma has indistinct margins. Mucinous carcinomas may appear as a high- or low-density mass on mammography based on the amount of extracellular mucinous component. Tumors with less cellularity and abundant mucin may have low density. Microcalcifications can be detected mammographically in 40% of cases and are

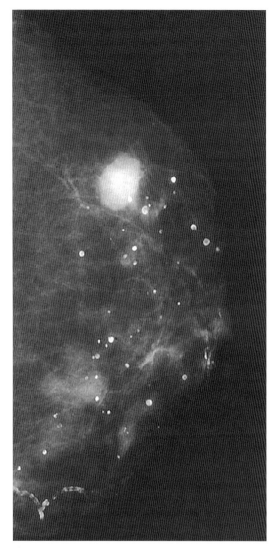

Fig. 9. **Mucinous carcinoma.** Mediolateral oblique mammographic image demonstrates a partially circumscribed, round, high-density left breast mass. Linear vascular and coarse calcifications are also present.

more commonly seen in a concurrent in situ carcinoma component or mucocele-like lesion.[34] Ultrasonographically, mucinous carcinoma presents as a complex solid and cystic mass that can be isoechoic or hypoechoic (see **Fig. 10**).

Gross Features

On gross examination, pure mucinous carcinomas form well circumscribed masses with a soft, mucinous consistency (**Figs. 11 and 12**).[12,13]

Key Features
MUCINOUS CARCINOMA

1. Large amount of extracellular mucin accumulation around nests of tumor cells

2. Low–to-intermediate tumor nuclear grade

3. Low tumor proliferative fraction

4. Absence of myoepithelial cells around tumor nests floating in mucin

5. Thin fibrovascular septa in mucin pools

6. Tumor cells positive for estrogen and progesterone receptors

7. Excellent prognosis

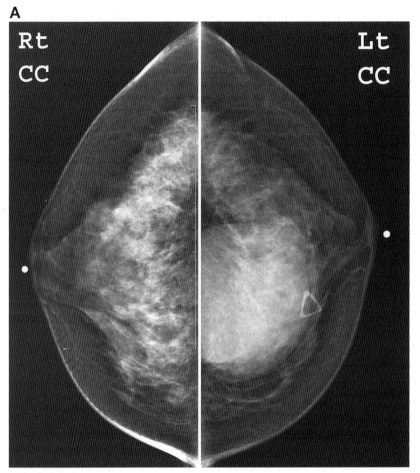

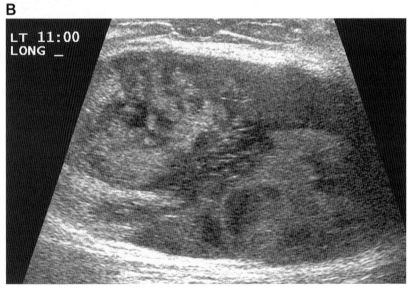

Fig. 10. (*A*) **Mucinous carcinoma**. A craniocaudal mammogram shows a large, round, high-density mass with partially obscured borders. (*B*) Mucinous carcinoma, ultrasonographic appearance. The well-circumscribed carcinoma is seen as a hypoechoic, septated, solid mass at ultrasound exhibiting enhanced through-transmission. A fibroepithelial lesion might be considered in the differential diagnosis, but because of the penetrating vessels, a cyst of any type would not be a consideration.

Fig.   11. **Mucinous carcinoma**.   (*A*)   Gross appearance of a small mucinous carcinoma. The tumor consists of many cystic nodules containing gray-white gelatinous substance. (*B*) Characteristic microscopic appearance   of   mucinous carcinoma. Small nests and clusters of uniform tumor cells float in mucin. Note the presence of thin fibrovascular   septae within the mucin pool (*arrows*). (*C*)   Higher magnification shows that tumor   clusters   are composed of monotonous tumor cells with round to oval nuclei. Mitotic figures are not easily identified.

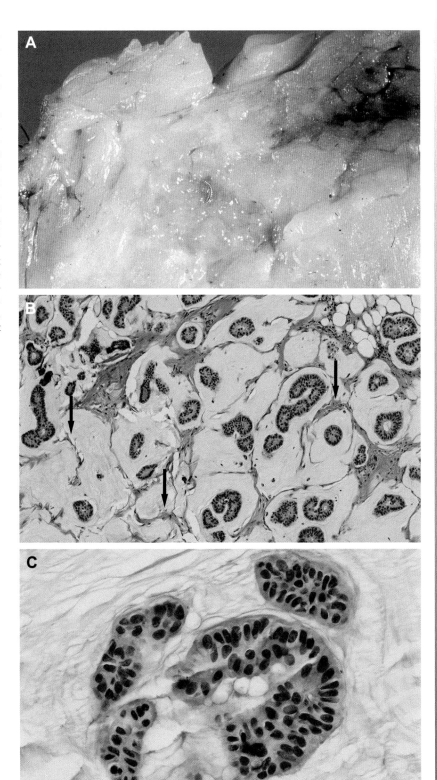

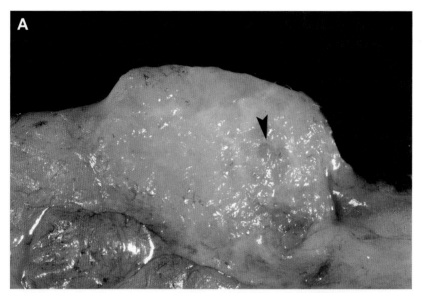

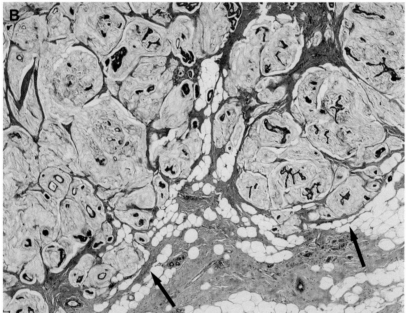

Fig. 12. **Mucinous carcinoma**. (*A*) Gross appearance, the tumor has well-circumscribed, lobulated contours and a gelatinous, gray-white cut surface. Small cystic spaces can be identified (*arrowhead*); (*B*) The lobulated growth pattern can also be seen and the margins are well-circumscribed. The tumor nests show knobby protrusion into adipose tissue (*arrows*).

Mixed mucinous carcinomas show a less distinct margin. The size is reported to range from 1 to 20 cm in the literature.[12,26–30] Older reports have indicated that mucinous carcinomas tend to be larger than conventional ductal carcinomas; however, more recent series have not shown any size difference between mucinous and nonmucinous carcinomas.[26,28]

Microscopic Features

Extracellular mucin pools containing tumor cells are the hallmark of mucinous carcinoma[12,13] (see **Fig. 11**). The amount of extracellular mucin and tumor cellularity varies, with some tumors being composed primarily of extracellular mucin with only a few clusters of tumor cells, and others

Fig. 13. **Mucinous carcinoma, hypocellular variant**. The tumor consists predominantly of pools of mucin. Only a few small tumor clusters are evident (*arrows*).

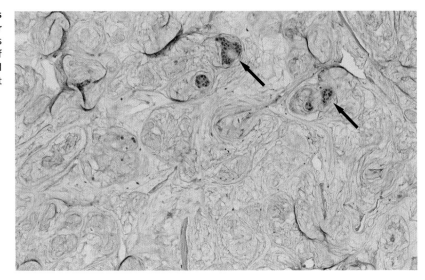

showing more tumor cells with less extracellular mucin (**Figs. 13** and **14**). The tumor cells are usually aggregated into small nests or papillary clusters, but may show a variety of growth patterns, including acini and tubule formation, alveolar nests and large nests with either solid growth or cribriform architecture (**Fig. 15**) (see also **Figs. 11** and **14**). The tumor cells are typically bland-looking with a low-to-intermediate nuclear grade (see **Fig. 11**). Mitoses are not frequently encountered.

If a cytologically high-grade carcinoma component is present in mucinous carcinoma, the tumor most likely represents a mixed mucinous

Fig. 14. **Mucinous carcinoma. hypercellular variant**. Varying sizes of nests and clusters of tumor cells are surrounded by mucin.

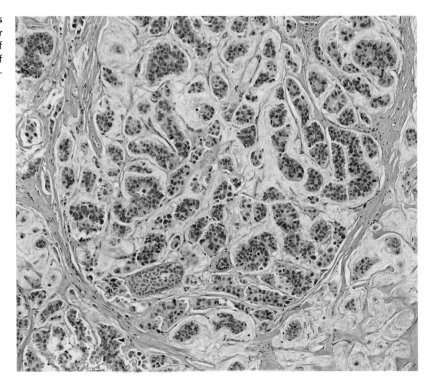

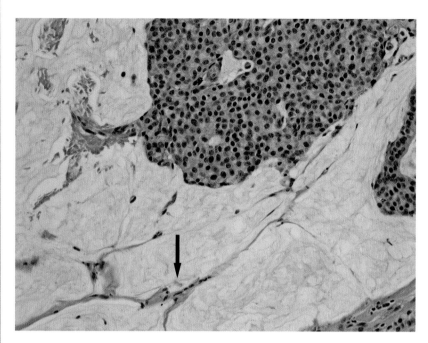

Fig. 15. **Mucinous carcinoma**. The tumor cells in mucinous carcinoma may grow in a variety of patterns, including a solid pattern. Thin fibrovascular septae are present in the extracellular mucin pool (*arrow*).

carcinoma and should not be classified as pure mucinous carcinoma.[35,36] No myoepithelial cells are found around the tumor clusters, which can be demonstrated by immunohistochemical analysis and can be used in the differential diagnosis of benign and malignant mucinous lesions. An in situ carcinoma component is present in the surrounding breast parenchyma in 30%–75% of mucinous carcinomas.[12,13,36] In the majority of cases, the in situ carcinoma component is low-to-intermediate grade carcinoma. Neuroendocrine differentiation has been described in mucinous carcinoma.[37,38] Some authors have suggested that mucinous carcinomas can be subclassified into types A, B, or AB on the basis of tumor cellularity and the presence of neuroendocrine differentiation.[38] Type A corresponds to classic mucinous carcinoma with predominantly extracellular mucin; type B corresponds to a variant of mucinous carcinoma showing neuroendocrine differentiation; type AB is considered to be an intermediate category. The biologic and clinical significance of this classification is still controversial. Thin fibrovascular septa may be present in the mucin pools, which is an important differential criterion because mucin pools in benign mucinous lesions are devoid of fibrovascular septa.

Mixed mucinous carcinomas are defined as carcinomas with a 50%–90% mucinous

carcinoma component. (**Fig. 16**) Mucinous differentiation is a relatively common finding in many invasive carcinomas of the breast, including invasive ductal and lobular carcinoma. To make a diagnosis of pure mucinous carcinoma, more than 90% of a tumor must be classic-type mucinous carcinoma.[12,13] The clinicopathologic features of mixed tumors are similar to those of conventional invasive ductal carcinoma.

Micropapillary differentiation has been described in mucinous carcinomas. Invasive micropapillary carcinomas of the breast are highly angioinvasive tumors.[12,13] The prognostic significance of the presence of focal micropapillary component in mucinous carcinomas has been controversial.[39,40]

Histochemically, the extracellular mucinous component of mucinous carcinoma is composed of acylated forms of sialomucins. Unlike gastrointestinal mucinous carcinoma cells, breast mucinous carcinoma cells contain only a small amount of neutral or acidic mucin.[9] Although studies on the expression of mucin genes and gene products have shown variable results in breast cancers, several studies have demonstrated that mucinous carcinomas of the breast typically show increased MUC2 and MUC5 overexpression (**Fig. 17**).[41,42] This is in contrast to conventional invasive ductal carcinomas, which

Fig. 16. **Mixed mucinous and ductal carcinoma.** Nonmucinous carcinoma is present (*left*) next to classic mucinous carcinoma.

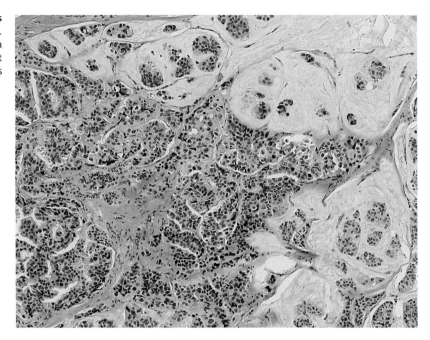

show frequent MUC1 overexpression. MUC2 and MUC5 overexpression is reported in less than 10% of nonmucinous breast cancers.

A high proportion of mucinous breast cancer is positive for estrogen and progesterone receptors. Published series have reported that 90% and 80% of mucinous carcinomas are positive for estrogen and progesterone receptors, respectively

(**Fig. 18**).[12,13,43] Her-2/neu overexpression and gene amplification is observed in less than 5% of mucinous carcinomas.[12,44]

Recently, gene expression profiling studies suggested a molecular subclassification of breast cancers distinguishing three major subtypes, luminal, basal-like, and Her-2/neu–positive breast cancers, which are characterized by distinct

Fig. 17. **Immunohistochemical staining for MUC-2.** Mucinous carcinoma cells showing diffuse cytoplasmic staining.

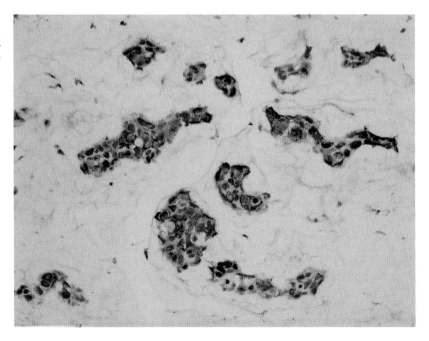

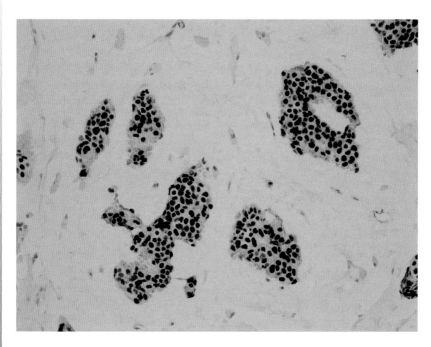

Fig. 18. **Immunohistochemical staining for estrogen receptor.** Diffuse nuclear positivity is present in tumor nuclei.

transcriptomic features and, most significantly, clinical outcomes. Limited data are available on molecular subtyping of special types of breast cancers including the mucinous carcinoma. In a recent investigation, Weigelt and colleagues[45] studied a series of 11 different histologic special-type breast carcinomas by immunohistochemistry and gene expression profiling. Mucinous carcinomas included in the study were classified as mucinous type A and mucinous type B tumors based on neuroendocrine differentiation. All mucinous carcinomas showed high similarity in overall gene expression, and were of luminal molecular subtype. In addition, they identified gene networks of invasion and proliferation to be down-regulated in mucinous type B tumors.[45] Similarly, Fujii and colleagues[46] evaluated the extent of loss of heterozygosity (LOH) in a group of mucinous carcinomas and compared the results with conventional invasive ductal carcinoma. They found an average frequency of LOH of only 1.9 of the 12 chromosomal arms in 18 cases of mucinous carcinoma, compared with an average frequency of LOH of 6.4 of these same chromosomal arms in cases of invasive ductal carcinoma. In three of the 18 cases of mucinous carcinoma studied, including one case with regional lymph node metastases, no LOH was seen at any of the 12 chromosomal regions studied. They concluded that mucinous cancers most likely have less genetic instability than most other forms of breast cancer and the

molecular pathogenesis of this form of breast cancer is likely to be substantially different than that of conventional ductal breast cancer.[46] The Wilms' tumor suppressor gene encodes a protein, WT1, that functions as a transcription regulator. Studies have suggested that immunohistochemical staining for WT1 is a good marker to differentiate between ovarian and peritoneal serous papillary carcinomas and breast carcinomas.[47] Although the majority of conventional invasive ductal carcinomas are negative for WT1 expression, up to two-thirds of pure mucinous carcinomas and one-third of mixed mucinous carcinomas have been reported to be positive for WT1.[48,49]

Differential Diagnosis

When a mucinous carcinoma is composed mostly of extracellular mucin pools with only a small number of tumor cells present, it may be difficult to differentiate from a mucocele-like lesion, especially with a limited sample such as a core biopsy. In such cases, identification of floating tumor cells in mucin pools is important and may require obtaining multiple deeper levels. Sometimes strips of epithelial lining of benign cyst or hyperplastic epithelium may be present in mucin pools; in such cases, the presence or absence of myoepithelial cells should be evaluated. Epithelial clusters lack myoepithelial cells in mucinous carcinoma. Identification of thin fibrovascular septa in mucin pools favors a diagnosis of mucinous carcinoma. The presence of epithelial cell nests sets apart mucinous carcinoma from other stromal lesions with a mucinous component such as myxoma, mucinosis, and mucinous degeneration after chemotherapy. Invasive lobular carcinoma with prominent signet ring cells may focally demonstrate areas of extracellular mucin, which may be confused with mucinous carcinoma with signet ring cells. However, mucinous carcinoma contains more prominent extracellular mucin pools and a smaller number of signet ring cells. Metastatic carcinoma to the breast from a gastrointestinal primary, including signet ring cell carcinoma, may be indistinguishable from mucinous carcinoma of the breast. In this case, the clinical presentation, the presence of an in situ carcinoma component, and an immunohistochemical profile of the tumor can be helpful in diagnosis.[12,13] Immunohistochemical staining for cytokeratin-7 and -20, estrogen and progesterone receptors, caudal-related homeobox gene 2 (CDX2), is most helpful. Mucinous carcinomas of the breast are positive for cytokeratin-7 and estrogen and progesterone receptors and are negative for cytokeratin-20 and CDX2; in contrast, gastrointestinal tract tumors are positive for cytokeratin-20 and CDX2 and are negative for cytokeratin-7 and estrogen and progesterone receptors. Metaplastic carcinomas may demonstrate mucinous/myxoid stromal changes, but other typical features such as squamous and mesenchymal differentiation and high-grade nuclear features are not observed in mucinous carcinoma.[50] Matrix-producing carcinoma is a subtype of metaplastic carcinoma of the breast and is characterized by an admixture of ductal carcinoma and mesenchymal matrix. The ductal carcinoma component is frequently high grade and the matrix is commonly chondromyxoid and may mimic mucinous material (**Fig. 19**). Other matrix-producing lesions such as mixed tumor of the breast (pleomorphic adenoma) may enter into differential diagnosis (**Fig. 20**) Centrally necrotizing breast cancer, characterized by an unusual and aggressive natural history, is composed of well-circumscribed, unicentric nodules with extensive central necrosis surrounded by a narrow rim of viable high-grade tumor cells, and may mimic mucinous carcinoma because the central necrosis may appear mucoid on low magnification view (**Fig. 21**). Mesenchymal lesions that produce myxoid stroma, such as myxoid sarcomas, are also in the differential diagnosis. Lack of epithelial clusters and more spindle appearance of cellular components should be helpful in this differential (**Fig. 22**). Immunohistochemical staining for cytokeratin can easily solve this differential, because mucinous carcinomas are diffusely positive for cytokeratin, whereas mesenchymal lesions are either totally negative or show very focal positivity.

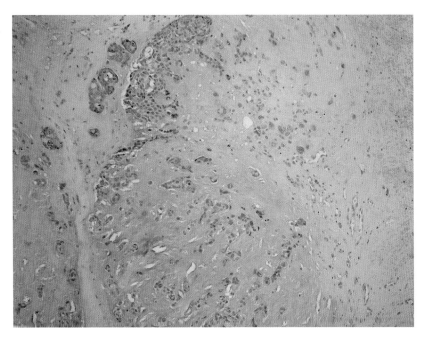

Fig. 19. **Matrix-producing carcinoma**. Chondromyxoid matrix.

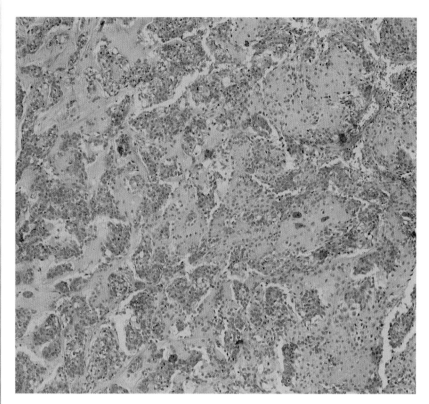

Fig. 20. **Pleomorphic adenoma**. Mixed tumor of the breast composed of variably sized epithelial cell nests admixed with chondromyxoid stroma. Calcification with ossification can be seen.

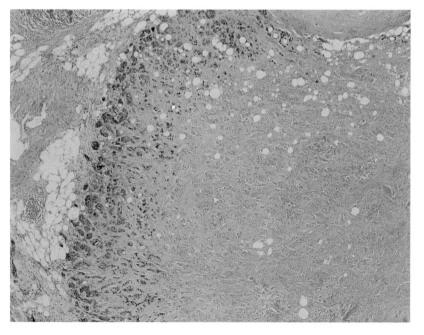

Fig. 21. **Centrally necrotizing breast cancer**. High-grade carcinoma. Note that tumor cells coalesce at the periphery and do not float in the mucin.

Fig. 22. **Myxoid sarcoma**. Proliferation of spindle cells in a background of myxoid stroma.

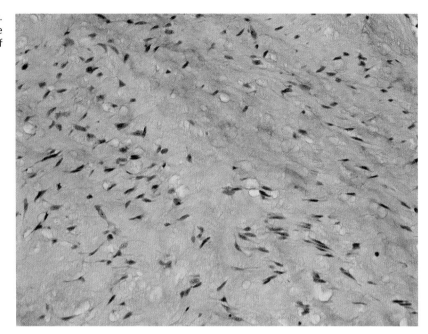

Prognosis

Patients who have pure mucinous carcinoma have a lower incidence of axillary lymph node metastasis, local and distant recurrences, and overall better clinical outcome compared with those who have conventional invasive ductal carcinoma. In a recent retrospective long-term follow-up study of 11,422 subjects who had mucinous carcinoma, the 10-, 15- and 20-year survival rates for mucinous carcinoma were 89%, 85%, and 81% respectively, compared with72%, 66%, and 62% for invasive ductal carcinoma.[26] Axillary lymph node metastasis occurs in less than 20% of cases of pure mucinous carcinoma. In the study by Barkley and colleagues,[27] no subjects with tumor size less than 1 cm had lymph node metastasis. When axillary lymph node involvement is present, usually a few lymph nodes are involved, and metastases may or may not have mucinous differentiation.[26–28,51] Distant metastases have been reported, and the pattern of metastases is similar to that of conventional ductal carcinoma. Mucinous carcinoma is a slow-growing neoplasm, and late systemic metastases have been reported. Established prognostic markers that are relevant for all other types of breast cancer also apply to mucinous breast cancer. Similar to all other types of breast cancers, axillary lymph node status is the most important predictor of clinical outcome.[12,13]

MUCINOUS CYSTADENOCARCINOMA

Mucinous cystadenocarcinoma is an extremely rare breast neoplasm reported predominantly in elderly women.[52–54] It resembles mucinous cystadenocarcinoma of the ovary and pancreas, and the tumor is reported to be composed of cystic spaces containing mucin and lined by tall columnar cells with intracellular mucin. Although none of the reported patients died of mucinous cystadenocarcinoma, evaluation of additional cases is necessary to further define the biologic behavior of this tumor. The absence of extracellular mucin pools containing tumor cells, and the presence of intracellular mucin, sets this tumor apart from mucinous carcinoma.

METASTATIC CARCINOMA

Metastasis to the breast from an extramammary site is uncommon.[55,56] Although malignant melanoma and hematologic malignancies are the most common primary tumors that are involved in such metastases, lung, stomach, and ovary have also been reported as frequent primary sites; metastasis from the colon, kidneys, uterine cervix, and thyroid have been reported to be even rarer.[57–59] Metastatic tumors usually present as small, painless, discrete nodules. Metastatic mucinous carcinomas may be histologically indistinguishable from mucinous carcinoma of the breast. The clinical presentation, the presence of an in situ carcinoma component, and the use of a panel of immunoantibodies may be helpful in establishing the diagnosis.[12,13]

BREAST LESIONS ASSOCIATED WITH INTRACELLULAR MUCIN PRODUCTION

Two distinct lesions of the breast demonstrate intracellular mucin: signet ring cell carcinoma and mucoepidermal carcinoma.

SIGNET RING CELL CARCINOMA

Signet ring cells are characterized by intracytoplasmic mucin accumulation and a crescent-shaped nucleus displaced toward one end of the cell. Primary breast cancers composed purely of signet ring cells are very rare and are not recognized as a separate entity of the World Health Organization classification.[36] Signet ring cell carcinoma of the breast is usually considered to be a variant of invasive lobular carcinoma; however, it can also be seen in association with invasive ductal carcinoma and mucinous carcinoma.[36,60]

Gross Features

Clinical presentation, imaging findings, and gross appearance of signet ring cell carcinoma are similar to those of conventional invasive ductal carcinoma.

Microscopic Features

Signet ring cell carcinoma cells are typically small, uniform, and dissociated; they are composed of a clear, vacuolated cytoplasm and have a compressed nucleus situated at the base of the cells (**Figs. 23** and **24**). The intracytoplasmic

---

Key Features
SIGNET RING CELL CARCINOMA OF BREAST

1. Abundant intracytoplasmic mucin accumulation with compression of the nucleus toward one pole of the cell

2. In most cases, the cells assume invasive lobular carcinoma growth pattern

3. May be associated with other types of invasive carcinoma

4. Associated with aggressive clinical behavior

5. Metastases to serosal surfaces common

---

mucin in signet ring cell carcinoma appears as a discrete secretion, which can be demonstrated with mucicarmine and Alcian blue stains. Although the number and percentage of signet ring cells required for diagnosis of signet ring cell carcinoma varies, most investigators diagnose signet ring cell carcinoma when at least 20% of tumor cells show signet ring cell morphology.[12,13,61] Because of its distinct morphology and aggressive clinical behavior, signet ring cell carcinoma should be noted when present and the percentage of signet ring cell differentiation needs to be mentioned.

Prognosis

Most reports suggest that the presence of a signet ring cell carcinoma component in invasive cancer imparts aggressive clinical behavior and an unusual metastatic pattern. Metastases to serosal surfaces such as the gastrointestinal tract, urinary bladder, uterus, and leptomeninges are frequent findings.[13]

Differential Diagnosis

Metastatic adenocarcinoma with signet ring cell features is the main differential diagnosis. When a breast tumor shows a predominantly pure signet ring cell carcinoma morphology, a metastatic tumor, especially from the gastrointestinal tract or the lung, should be excluded. Identification of an in situ carcinoma component is the most important finding to differentiate primary versus metastatic signet ring cell carcinoma. The presence of more typical breast carcinoma infiltration patterns is also suggestive of the primary nature of this tumor. Many studies have evaluated immunohistochemical profiles of signet ring cell carcinomas of different organ sites. Signet ring cell carcinomas of the breast are positive for cytokeratin-7 and negative for cytokeratin-20.[61–63] Estrogen and progesterone receptors are frequently expressed in signet ring cell carcinomas of the breast. The mucin profiles for gastric, colorectal, and breast signet ring cell carcinomas are reported to have distinct mucin expression patterns that are maintained in metastases.[62] Mucin profiling may be useful to identify the origin of a metastatic signet ring cell carcinoma of unknown primary. Signet ring cell breast cancers are typically positive for MUC1, weakly positive for MUC2, 5, and 6, and negative for MUC4.[63] In a recent study, Sentani and colleagues[64] reported Reg IV and claudin immunohistochemical staining patterns of signet ring carcinoma from different organ sites. All cases of gastric and colorectal signet ring cell carcinomas were positive for Reg IV, and all the remaining signet ring cell carcinomas, including breast carcinomas, were negative. Eighty-six

Fig. 23. **Signet ring cell carcinoma**. (*A*) Low magnification showing diffuse infiltration of signet ring cells. (*B*) High magnification of signet ring cells showing intracellular mucin and compressed peripheral nucleus.

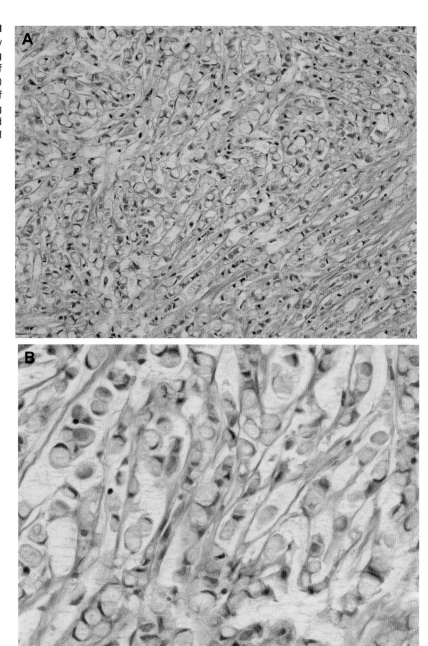

percent of gastric and 38% of colorectal signet ring cell carcinomas were positive for claudin-18, whereas all other signet ring cell carcinomas were negative. The authors concluded that Reg IV staining and claudin-18 staining can aid in diagnosis of gastrointestinal signet ring cell carcinomas.[64]

Both lipid-rich and glycogen-rich carcinomas of the breast may have cytoplasmic vacuoles that may mimic signet ring cell carcinoma. As the names imply, tumor cells have abundant lipid and glycogen in lipid-rich[65] and glycogen-rich[66] carcinomas, respectively. The presence of lipid and glycogen in these tumors can be

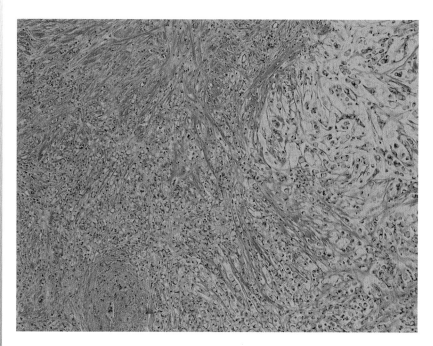

Fig. 24. **Signet ring cell carcinoma.** Signet ring cell carcinoma showing focal extracellular mucinous accumulation.

demonstrated by special histochemical stains (mucicarmine, periodic acid–Schiff, and oil red O). Additionally, electron microscopy may be useful in differentiating them from signet ring cell carcinomas.

MUCOEPIDERMOID CARCINOMA

Mucoepidermoid carcinoma of the breast is a rare tumor occurring predominantly in postmenopausal women (mean age, 55 years) and resembles mucoepidermoid carcinoma of the salivary gland.[67] Histologically, it is composed of cystic and solid areas and consists of various cell types including basaloid, intermediate, mucinous, and squamoid cells. The majority of reported cases have had a very aggressive course with early recurrences and poor outcome. The absence of extracellular mucin pools containing tumor cells, and the presence of intracellular mucin and squamoid cells, sets this tumor apart from mucinous carcinoma.

BREAST LESIONS ASSOCIATED WITH BOTH INTRACELLULAR AND EXTRACELLULAR MUCIN PRODUCTION

Two uncommon types of breast lesions demonstrate both intra- and extracellular mucin: secretory carcinoma and adenoid cystic carcinoma.

SECRETORY CARCINOMA

Secretory carcinoma of the breast is an uncommon and distinct type of breast cancer that was first described in children. Although it most commonly occurs in children and young adults (under 30 years), occasionally it occurs in older women.[68,69] Molecular analyses have shown that secretory carcinoma cells have an ETV6–NTRK3 fusion gene, which is a distinctive genetic abnormality also seen in pediatric mesenchymal tumors.[70]

Gross Features

Typically, secretory carcinomas form a well-circumscribed, firm, lobulated mass that is commonly located near the areola. The tumors tend to be smaller than 2 cm.

Microscopic Features

Secretory carcinoma is characterized by lobulated and well-defined margins. The tumor cells form irregular tubular, papillary, cystic, and solid structures containing abundant intracellular and extracellular secretory material (**Fig. 25**). The extracellular secretions are densely eosinophilic and positive for periodic acid–Schiff reaction after diastase digestion. The intracellular secretions may show variable reactions to mucins and periodic acid–Schiff stain. The tumor cells show minimal pleomorphism. Mitoses and necrosis are

Fig. 25. **Secretory carcinoma**. (*A*) Low magnification showing microcystic and macrocystic spaces containing abundant intraluminal secretory material. (*B*) High magnification showing that both solid and microcystic areas are composed of low-grade tumor cells.

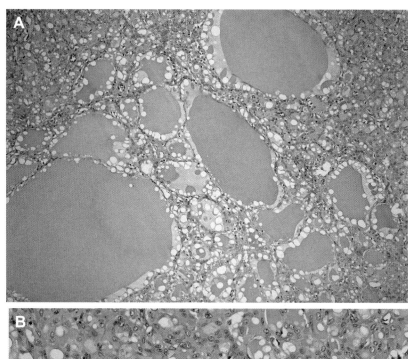

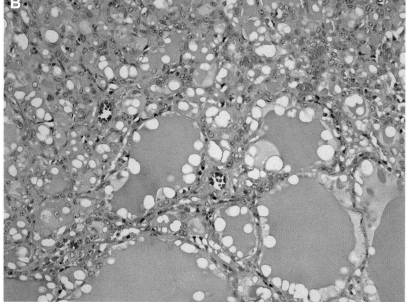

rarely observed. An in situ carcinoma component is usually reported.

have been reported but have rarely involved more than a few lymph nodes.

Prognosis

Secretory carcinoma has an extremely good prognosis in children and young adults; however, in older patients, it may have a more aggressive clinical behavior. Axillary lymph node metastases

Differential Diagnosis

Due to the presence of abundant intracellular and extracellular secretions, secretory carcinoma can be confused with other mucinous lesions of the breast, especially in limited samples.

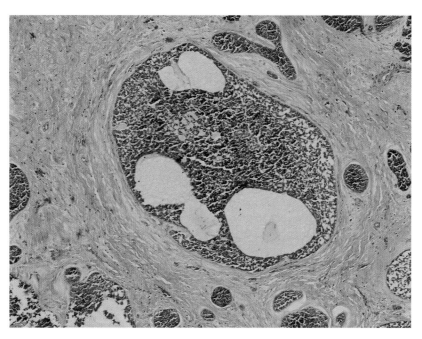

Fig. 26. Adenoid cystic carcinoma of the breast. Adenoid cystic carcinoma of breast showing solid and cribriform patterns. The intraluminal mucoid material in the cribriform areas may resemble mucinous carcinoma. The tumor cells are composed of basaloid cells.

ADENOID CYSTIC CARCINOMA

Adenoid cystic carcinoma is a rare form of invasive breast cancer accounting for less than 1% of all primary breast cancers.[71] The age distribution is similar to that of conventional invasive ductal carcinoma.

Gross Features

Typically adenoid cystic carcinoma forms a well-demarcated solid or cystic mass, typically less than 3 cm.[71,72]

Microscopic Features

The microscopic pattern of adenoid cystic carcinoma is variable, with cribriform, tubular, trabecular, and solid patterns (**Fig. 26**). Several of these patterns coexist in many cases. Tubular structures contain mucoid material that may be copious and in some cases may mimic mucinous carcinoma. Two cell types are present in adenoid cystic carcinoma: basaloid cells and cells with fibrillar, elongated cytoplasm. The stroma is hyalinized, and in some cases, this hyalinized stroma predominates and may mimic extracellular mucin pools seen in mucinous carcinomas. The majority of adenoid cystic carcinomas are negative for estrogen and progesterone receptors and Her-2/neu overexpression.[71]

Prognosis

Adenoid cystic carcinoma is one of the least aggressive neoplasms of the breast. Lymph node metastases are rare. Recurrences and rare distant metastases have been reported. Grading of adenoid cystic carcinoma of the breast using a grading system similar to that used for adenoid cystic carcinomas of salivary gland origin may be helpful in predicting aggressive clinical behavior.[71]

Differential Diagnosis

Invasive cribriform carcinoma,[36] invasive ductal carcinoma with cribriform features, mucinous carcinoma, and collagenous spherulosis[73] (**Fig. 27**) are the main differential diagnoses. Identification of two cell types in adenoid cystic carcinoma is the main clue to establishing the diagnosis. Unlike mucinous carcinoma, in which tumor cells float in mucin, extracellular secretions in adenoid cystic carcinoma are intraluminal. Collagenous spherulosis is a rare benign lesion that can microscopically mimic adenoid cystic carcinoma. Degenerative cystic changes with accumulation of secretions in collagenous spherulosis may mimic extracellular mucin production.

Fig.   27. **Collegenous spherulosis**. (*A*) Degenerative cystic changes with accumulation of secretions is shown in this benign lesion. (*B*) High magnification view shows the fibrillar nature of the material accumulated in each spherule.

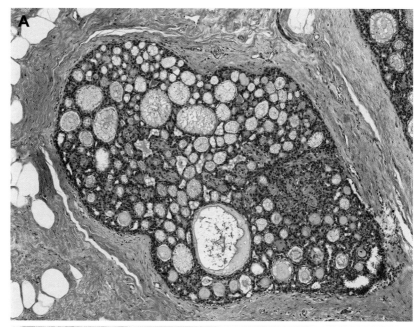

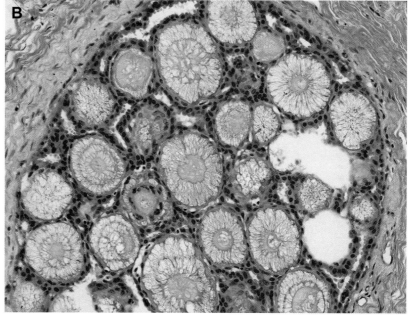

OTHER LESIONS ASSOCIATED WITH MUCIN PRODUCTION OR MIMICKING MUCIN

Connective tissue cells may also produce mucin or mucin-like substances and mimic mucinous lesions of the breast. Mucinous stroma has been described in fibroepithelial lesions including both fibroadenoma and phyllodes tumor.

Injected foreign substances may mimic extracellular mucin production and histiocytes containing foreign materials may mimic signet ring cell carcinoma. Foreign materials injected for breast augmentation or, more commonly, foreign substances injected into biopsy sites, may have a histologic appearance similar to that of mucin (**Figs. 28** and **29**).[74] The presence of a foreign

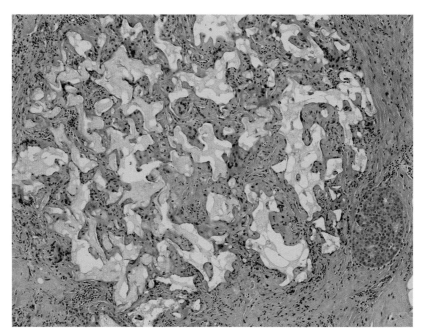

Fig. 28. Foreign material. Foreign material inserted during core needle biopsy may mimic extracellular mucin production. There is usually associated previous biopsy change.

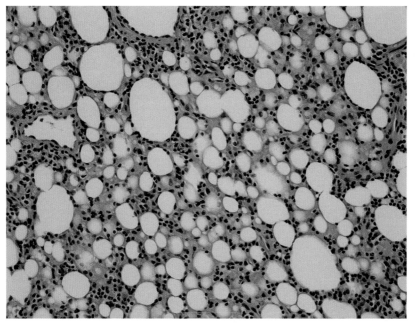

Fig. 29. Foreign material. The variable size of intracytoplasmic globules, identification of foreign material and presence of other inflammatory cells are helpful clues to diagnosis.

Table 2
Lesions with stromal substances that mimic mucin production

Neoplasm	Non-Neoplastic Lesions
Fibroepithelial lesions	Mucinosis
Salivary gland-like tumors	Biopsy site changes
Pleomorphic adenoma (mixed tumor)	Post-therapy changes
Metaplastic carcinoma	Foreign material
Centrally necrotizing carcinoma	
Mesenchymal neoplasms	
Myxoma	
Myxoid sarcoma	

Pitfalls
MUCINOUS LESIONS OF BREAST

Acellular mucin

! Mucinous carcinomas can be hypocellular and may appear as acellular mucin. Examination of multiple deeper levels may be necessary to demonstrate epithelial clusters.

! Any type of epithelial proliferations may be associated with extracellular mucin spillage into stroma.

! Simple cysts may rupture and dissect into stroma.

Myxoid Stromal Changes

! Myxoid changes in benign neoplasms such as fibroadenoma may mimic mucinous lesions.

! Neoplasms with fibromyxoid stromal changes such as salivary gland-like tumors may mimic lesions.

Mucin-Like Material

Extracellular

  ! Foreign bodies related to biopsy may mimic mucin

  ! Stromal hyalinization may appear as mucin

  ! Necrosis may mimic mucin

Intracellular

  ! Glycogen-rich carcinoma

  ! Apocrine carcinoma

  ! Lipid-rich carcinoma

  ! May mimic intracellular mucin production

body reaction and biopsy site changes can be helpful; in addition, the injected foreign materials may have different tinctorial qualities (**Table 2**).

REFERENCES

1. Perez-Vilar J, Hill RL. In: Lennarz, Lane, editors, Mucin family of glycoproteins. Encyclopedia of biological chemistry, vol. 2. Oxford (UK): Academic Press/Elsevier; 2004. p. 758–64.
2. Moniaux N, Escande F, Porchet N, et al. Structural organization and classification of the human mucin genes. Front Biosci 2001;6:D1192–206.
3. Ringel J, Lohr M. The MUC gene family: their role in diagnosis and early detection of pancreatic cancer. Mol Cancer 2003;7:2–9.
4. Singh PK, Hollingsworth MA. Cell surface-associated mucins in signal transduction. Trends Cell Biol 2006;16(9):467–76.
5. Gendler SJ, Lancaster CA, Taylor-Papadimitriou J, et al. Molecular cloning and expression of human tumour-associated polymorphic epithelial mucin. J Biol Chem 1990;265(25):15286–93.
6. Adsay NV, Merati K, Nassar H, et al. Pathogenesis of colloid (pure mucinous) carcinoma of exocrine organs: coupling of gel-forming mucin (MUC2) production with altered cell polarity and abnormal cell-stroma interaction may be the key factor in the morphogenesis and indolent behavior of colloid carcinoma in the breast and pancreas. Am J Surg Pathol 2003;27(5):571–8.
7. Hanna WM, Corkill M. Mucins in breast carcinoma. Hum Pathol 1988;19(1):11–4.
8. Tan PH, Tse GM, Bay BH. Mucinous breast lesions: diagnostic challenges. J Clin Pathol 2008;61(1): 11–9.
9. Chinyama CN, Davies JD. Mammary mucinous lesions: congeners, prevalence and important pathological associations. Histopathology 1996;29(6): 533–9.

10. Weaver MG, Abdul-Karim FW, al-Kaisi N. Mucinous lesions of the breast. A pathological continuum. Pathol Res Pract 1993;189(8):873–6.

11. Cooper DJ. Mucin histochemistry of mucous carcinomas of breast and colon and non-neoplastic breast epithelium. J Clin Pathol 1974;27(4):311–4.

12. Rosen PP. Rosen's breast pathology. 3rd edition. Philadelphia: Lippincott Williams and Wilkins; 2008.

13. Tavassoli FA. Pathology of the breast. 2nd edition. Stanford (CT): Appleton & Lange; 1999.

14. Rosen PP. Mucocele-like tumors of the breast. Am J Surg Pathol 1986;10(7):464–9.

15. Ro JY, Sneige N, Sahin AA, et al. Mucocelelike tumor of the breast associated with atypical ductal hyperplasia or mucinous carcinoma. A clinicopathologic study of seven cases. Arch Pathol Lab Med 1991; 115(2):137–40.

16. Hamele-Bena D, Cranor ML, Rosen PP. Mammary mucocele-like lesions. Benign and malignant. Am J Surg Pathol 1996;20(9):1081–5.

17. Coyne JD. Columnar cell hyperplasia with intraluminal crystalloids and features of a mucocele-like lesion. Histopathology 2004;44(4):401–3.

18. Fadare O, Mariappan MR. Mucocele-like tumor and columnar cell hyperplasia of the breast occurring in a morphologic continuum. J Med Case Reports 2008;2:138–41.

19. Tanaka K, Komoike Y, Egawa C, et al. Indeterminate calcification and clustered cystic lesions are strongly predictive of the presence of mucocele-like tumor of the breast: a report of six cases. Breast Cancer 2009;16(1):77–82.

20. Farshid G, Pieterse S, King JM, et al. Mucocele-like lesions of the breast: a benign cause for indeterminate or suspicious mammographic microcalcifications. Breast J 2005;11(1):15–22.

21. Simsir A, Tsang P, Greenebaum E. Additional mimics of mucinous mammary carcinoma: fibroepithelial lesions. Am J Clin Pathol 1998;109(2):169–72.

22. Sanati S, Leonard M, Khamapirad T, et al. Nodular mucinosis of the breast: a case report with pathologic, ultrasonographic, and clinical findings and review of the literature. Arch Pathol Lab Med 2005;129(3):e58–61.

23. Balci P, Kabakci N, Topcu I, et al. Breast myxoma: radiologic and histopathologic features. Breast J 2007;13(1):88–90.

24. Carder PJ, Murphy CE, Liston JC. Surgical excision is warranted following a core biopsy diagnosis of mucocele-like lesion of the breast. Histopathology 2004;45(2):148–54.

25. Wang J, Simsir A, Mercado C, et al. Can core biopsy reliably diagnose mucinous lesions of the breast? Am J Clin Pathol 2007;127(1):124–7.

26. Di Saverio S, Gutierrez J, Avisar E. A retrospective review with long term follow up of 11,400 cases of pure mucinous breast carcinoma. Breast Cancer Res Treat 2008;111(3):541–7.

27. Barkley CR, Ligibel JA, Wong JS, et al. Mucinous breast carcinoma: a large contemporary series. Am J Surg 2008;196(4):549–51.

28. Komenaka IK, El-Tamer MB, Troxel A, et al. Pure mucinous carcinoma of the breast. Am J Surg 2004;187(4):528–32.

29. Lannigan AK, Going JJ, Weiler-Mithoff E, et al. Mucinous breast carcinoma. Breast 2002;11(4): 359–61.

30. Andre S, Cunha F, Bernardo M, et al. Mucinous carcinoma of the breast: a pathologic study of 82 cases. J Surg Oncol 1995;58(3):162–7.

31. Clayton F. Pure mucinous carcinomas of breast: morphologic features and prognostic correlates. Hum Pathol 1986;17(1):34–8.

32. Toikkanen S, Kujari H. Pure and mixed mucinous carcinomas of the breast: a clinicopathologic analysis of 61 cases with long-term follow-up. Hum Pathol 1989;20(8):758–64.

33. Matsuda M, Yoshimoto M, Iwase T, et al. Mammographic and clinicopathological features of mucinous carcinoma of the breast. Breast Cancer 2000;7(1):65–70.

34. Wilson TE, Helvie MA, Oberman HA, et al. Pure and mixed mucinous carcinoma of the breast: pathologic basis for differences in mammographic appearance. AJR Am J Roentgenol 1995;165(2): 285–9.

35. NHS Breast Screening Programme. Pathology Reporting of Breast Disease. NHS Breast Screening Programme, publication number 58:2005.

36. Tavassoli FA, Devilee P. World Health Organization Classification of Tumours. Pathology and genetics of tumours of the breast and female genital organs. Lyon (France): IARC Press; 2003.

37. Kato N, Endo Y, Tamura G, et al. Mucinous carcinoma of the breast: a multifaceted study with special reference to histogenesis and neuroendocrine differentiation. Pathol Int 1999;49(11):947–55.

38. Scopsi L, Andreola S, Pilotti S, et al. Mucinous carcinoma of the breast. A clinicopathologic, histochemical and immunocytochemical study with special reference to neuroendocrine differentiation. Am J Surg Pathol 1994;18(7):702–11.

39. Shet T, Chinoy R. Presence of a micropapillary pattern in mucinous carcinomas of the breast and its impact on the clinical behavior. Breast J 2008; 14(5):412–20.

40. Bal A, Joshi K, Sharma SC, et al. Prognostic significance of micropapillary pattern in pure mucinous carcinoma of the breast. Int J Surg Pathol 2008; 16(3):251–6.

41. Matsukita S, Nomoto M, Kitajima S, et al. Expression of mucins (MUC1, MUC2, MUC5AC and MUC6) in mucinous carcinoma of the breast: comparison with invasive ductal carcinoma. Histopathology 2003;42(1):26–36.

42. Rakha EA, Boyce RW, Abd El-Rehim D, et al. Expression of mucins (MUC1, MUC2, MUC3, MUC4, MUC5AC and MUC6) and their prognostic significance in human breast cancer. Mod Pathol 2005;18(10):1295–304.

43. Cho LC, Hsu YH. Expression of androgen, estrogen and progesterone receptors in mucinous carcinoma of the breast. Kaohsiung J Med Sci 2008;24(5):227–32.

44. Bilous M, Ades C, Armes J, et al. Predicting the HER2 status of breast cancer from basic histopathology data: an analysis of 1500 breast cancers as part of the HER2000 International Study. Breast 2003;12(2):92–8.

45. Weigelt B, Horlings HM, Kreike B, et al. Refinement of breast cancer classification by molecular characterization of histological special types. J Pathol 2008;216(2):141–50.

46. Fujii H, Anbazhagan R, Bornman DM, et al. Mucinous cancers have fewer genomic alterations than more common classes of breast cancer. Breast Cancer Res Treat 2002;76(3):255–60.

47. Tornos C, Soslow R, Chen S, et al. Expression of WT1, CA 125, and GCDFP-15 as useful markers in the differential diagnosis of primary ovarian carcinomas versus metastatic breast cancer to the ovary. Am J Surg Pathol 2005;29(11):1482–9. Erratum in: Am J Surg Pathol 2006;Jan;30(1):140.

48. Domfeh AB, Carley AL, Striebel JM, et al. WT1 immunoreactivity in breast carcinoma: selective expression in pure and mixed mucinous subtypes. Mod Pathol 2008;21(10):1217–23.

49. Steinbrecher JS, Silverberg SG. Signet-ring cell carcinoma of the breast. The mucinous variant of infiltrating lobular carcinoma? Cancer 1976;37(2):828–40.

50. Pezzi CM, Patel-Parekh L, Cole K, et al. Characteristics and treatment of metaplastic breast cancer: analysis of 892 cases from the National Cancer Data Base. Ann Surg Oncol 2007;14(1):166–73.

51. Rasmussen BB. Human mucinous breast carcinoma and their lymph node metastases. A histological review of 247 cases. Pathol Res Pract 1985;180(4):377–82.

52. Koenig C, Tavassoli FA. Mucinous cystadenocarcinoma of the breast. Am J Surg Pathol 1998;22(6):698–703.

53. Chen WY, Chen CS, Chen HC, et al. Mucinous cystadenocarcinoma of the breast coexisting with infiltrating ductal carcinoma. Pathol Int 2004;54(10):781–6.

54. Lee SH, Chaung CR. Mucinous metaplasia of breast carcinoma with macrocystic transformation resembling ovarian mucinous cystadenocarcinoma in a case of synchronous bilateral infiltrating ductal carcinoma. Pathol Int 2008;58(9):601–5.

55. Georgiannos SN, Chin J, Goode AW, et al. Secondary neoplasms of the breast. A survey of the 20th Century. Cancer 2001;92(9):2259–66.

56. Nielsen M, Andersen JA, Henriksen FW, et al. Metastases to the breast from extramammary carcinomas. Acta Pathol Microbiol Scand [A] 1981;89(4):251–6.

57. Toombs BD, Kalisher L. Metastatic disease to the breast: clinical, pathologic and radiographic features. Am J Roentgenol 1977;129(4):673–6.

58. Magri K, Demoulin G, Millon G, et al. Metastasis to the breast from non mammary metastasis. Clinical, radiological characteristics and diagnostic process. A report of two cases and a review of literature. J Gynecol Obstet Biol Reprod (Paris) 2007;36(6):602–6.

59. Alexander HR, Turnbull AD, Rosen PP. Isolated breast metastases from gastrointestinal carcinomas: report of two cases. J Surg Oncol 1989;42(4):264–6.

60. Kuroda N, Fujishima N, Ohara M, et al. Invasive ductal carcinoma of the breast with signet-ring cell and mucinous carcinoma components: diagnostic utility of immunocytochemistry of signet-ring cells in aspiration cytology materials. Diagn Cytopathol 2007;35(3):171–3.

61. Raju U, Ma CK, Shaw A. Signet ring variant of lobular carcinoma of the breast: a clinicopathologic and immunohistochemical study. Mod Pathol 1993;6(5):516–20.

62. Nguyen MD, Plasil B, Wen P, et al. Mucin profiles in signet-ring cell carcinoma. Arch Pathol Lab Med 2006;130(6):799–804.

63. Chu PG, Schwarz RE, Lau SK, et al. Immunohistochemical staining in the diagnosis of pancreatobiliary and ampulla of Vater adenocarcinoma: application of CDX2, CK17, MUC1, and MUC2. Am J Surg Pathol 2005;29(3):359–67.

64. Sentani K, Oue N, Tashiro T, et al. Immunohistochemical staining of Reg IV and claudin-18 is useful in the diagnosis of gastrointestinal signet ring cell carcinoma. Am J Surg Pathol 2008;32(8):1182–9.

65. Dina R, Eusebi V. Clear cell tumors of the breast. Semin Diagn Pathol 1997;14(3):175–82.

66. Hayes MM, Seidman JD, Ashton MA. Glycogen-rich clear cell carcinoma of the breast. A clinicopathologic study of 21 cases. Am J Surg Pathol 1995;19(8):904–11.

67. Horii R, Akiyama F, Ikenaga M, et al. Muco-epidermoid carcinoma of the breast. Pathol Int 2006;56(9):549–53.

68. Diallo R, Tognon C, Knezevich SR, et al. Secretory carcinoma of the breast: a genetically defined carcinoma entity. Verh Dtsch Ges Pathol 2003;87:193–203.

69. Mun SH, Ko EY, Han BK, et al. Secretory carcinoma of the breast: sonographic features. J Ultrasound Med 2008;27(6):947–54.

70. Tognon C, Knezevich SR, Huntsman D, et al. Expression of the ETV6-NTRK3 gene fusion as a primary event in human secretory breast carcinoma. Cancer Cell 2002;2(5):367–76.

71. Soon SR, Yong WS, Ho GH, et al. Adenoid cystic breast carcinoma: a salivary gland-type tumour

with excellent prognosis and implications for management. Pathology 2008;40(4):413–5.

72. Pia-Foschini M, Reis-Filho JS, Eusebi V, et al. Salivary gland-like tumours of the breast: surgical and molecular pathology. J Clin Pathol 2003;56(7):497–506.

73. Resetkova E, Albarracin C, Sneige N. Collagenous spherulosis of breast: morphologic study of 59 cases and review of the literature. Am J Surg Pathol 2006;30(1):20–7.

74. Gould E, Perez J, Albores-Saavedra J, et al. Signet ring cell sinus histiocytosis. A previously unrecognized histologic condition mimicking metastatic carcinoma in lymph nodes. Am J Clin Pathol 1989; 92:509–12.

Index

Note: Page numbers of article titles are in **boldface** type.

A

Abscess, breast, squamous metaplasia of lactiferous ducts vs., 394

Adenocarcinoma, metastatic, with signet ring cell features, signet cell carcinoma vs., 431–432

Adenoid cystic carcinoma, 434
  differential diagnosis of, 435
  microscopic features of, 434
  prognosis for, 434
  vs. collagenous spherulosis, 435

Adenoma, of nipple, 397–400
    syringomatous, 403–404
    pleomorphic, mucinous carcinoma vs., 425, 429

Adenosis, ductal carcinoma, invasive, mimicking, 353

Adenosquamous carcinoma, p63 reactivity in, 356, 358
    smooth muscle myosin heavy chain immunostain in, 356, 357

Angiosarcoma, epithelioid, triple-negative carcinoma vs., 256

Apocrine lesions, flat epithelial atypia vs., 266–267

Atypical ductal hyperplasia (ADH), collagenous spherulosis mimicking, 242–243
  DCIS vs., 240, 242–243
  diagnosis on core biopsy, 244–245
  differential diagnosis of, 240–242
  flat epithelial atypia vs., 267–268
  flat epithelial atypia with, 270
  key features of, 236
  microscopic features of, 236, 240
    vs. low-grade DCIS, 236, 240

Atypical lobular hyperplasia (ALH), comparison with classical lobular carcinoma in situ, 285–287
  diagnosis of, 285
  immunoprofile of, 286–287
  markers for, cytokeratin 8, 287
    E-cadherin, 286
    estrogen receptor, 287
    high-molecular weight cytokeratin, 287
    P120 catenin for, 286–287
  microscopic features of, 285
  on core biopsy, classical lobular carcinoma in situ or ALH, 285–286
  prognosis in, 285

B

Basal-like carcinoma, gene expression profiling of, 256–257
  immunohistochemical studies of, 257

Breast cancer, centrally necrotizing, mucinous carcinoma vs., 425, 430

C

Calponin, in differential diagnosis of benign and invasive lesions, 352, 355
    in myoepithelial cell attenuation, 361
    in overlooked invasive foci, 358–359
    in tubular adenosis, 365, 367–368

CAM5.2, Toker cell immunoreactivity to, 404, 407

CD10, in differential diagnosis of benign and invasive lesions, 355

CD34, in myofibroblastoma, 384

CD117 (c-kit), for phyllodes tumor prognosis, 312

CK5/6, in encapsulated papillary carcinoma, 341

CK5/14, in encapsulated papillary carcinoma, 341

CK7, in lesions of nipple skin, 408
    Toker cell immunoreactivity to, 404, 407

CK8, in classical lobular carcinoma in situ, 287

CK19, in flat epithelial atypia, 265

Classical lobular carcinoma in situ (C-LCIS), as precursor to invasive lobular carcinoma, 285
    as risk lesion, 284–285
    associated lesions in, 273
    atrophy of terminal duct lobular units in, 277
    calcification in, 273
    differential diagnosis of, 277–278
    lesions mimicking, 278–279
    microscopic features of, acini, 275, 277
        and cloverleaf configuration of duct, 276, 279
        intracytoplastic vacuoles, 274–275
        pagetoid extension, 276, 279
        type A cells, 274, 276–277
        type B cells, 274, 276–277
    morphologic features of, 277, 280
    nonneoplastic proliferation mimicking severe lesion, collagenous spherulosis, 281–283
        sclerosing lesions, 280–281
        usual ductal hyperplasia, 283–284

Clear cell change, in TDLU, classical lobular carcinoma in situ vs., 279–280

Collagenous spherulosis, adenoid cystic carcinoma vs., 435

Columnar cell change, flat epithelial atypia vs., 266–267, 269

Columnar cell hyperplasia, flat epithelial atypia vs., 266–267, 269

Cystadenocarcinoma, mucinous, 427

Cystic hypersecretory hyperplasia (CHH), pregnancy-like, 266–268

Cyst(s), benign, 413, 414–415
    epidermal inclusion of nipple, 394

Cytokeratin immunostain, in in situ and invasive carcinoma, 364–365

doi:10.1016/S1875-9181(09)00027-0
1875-9181/09/$ – see front matter © 2009 Elsevier Inc. All rights reserved.

Moving?

Make sure your subscription moves with you!

To notify us of your new address, find your **Clinics Account Number** (located on your mailing label above your name), and contact customer service at:

E-mail: elspcs@elsevier.com

800-654-2452 (subscribers in the U.S. & Canada)
314-453-7041 (subscribers outside of the U.S. & Canada)

Fax number: 314-523-5170

Elsevier Periodicals Customer Service
11830 Westline Industrial Drive
St. Louis, MO 63146

*To ensure uninterrupted delivery of your subscription, please notify us at least 4 weeks in advance of move.

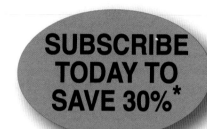
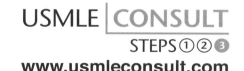